THE EVERYTHING
Guide to
Pregnancy Over 35

Dear Reader,

We wrote this book because we strongly believe that all women deserve to have, and can have, happy and healthy pregnancies, regardless of their age. Becoming a mother is one of the most exciting times in your life, but too often mothers who are over age 35 spend a lot of their time worrying about what could go wrong in their pregnancy. Being an over-35 mom should be about so much more.

Our goal in this book is not only to help you understand actual risks about the things you are concerned about, but also to set your mind at rest. Age is just one of many factors in pregnancy, and not many health-care providers even blink an eye at an older mother these days. Most women who are over age 35 are going to have healthy pregnancies and babies. As an older mom, you may face different challenges than younger moms, and we've tried to address everything that might be of concern to you. Congratulations on your pregnancy!

Brette M. Sember

Dr. Bruce D. Rodgers

Diane E. Rodgers, R.N.C.

The EVERYTHING® Series

Editorial

Innovation Director	Paula Munier
Editorial Director	Laura M. Daly
Executive Editor, Series Books	Brielle K. Matson
Associate Copy Chief	Sheila Zwiebel
Acquisitions Editor	Kerry Smith
Development Editor	Brett Palana-Shanahan
Production Editor	Casey Ebert

Production

Director of Manufacturing	Susan Beale
Production Project Manager	Michelle Roy Kelly
Prepress	Erick DaCosta
	Matt LeBlanc
Interior Layout	Heather Barrett
	Brewster Brownville
	Colleen Cunningham
	Jennifer Oliveira
Cover Design	Erin Alexander
	Stephanie Chrusz
	Frank Rivera

THE
EVERYTHING®
GUIDE TO PREGNANCY OVER 35

From conquering your fears to assessing
health risks—all you need to have a
happy, healthy nine months

Brette McWhorter Sember

Technical Review by Bruce D. Rodgers, M.D., and Diane E. Rodgers, R.N.C.

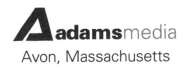

Avon, Massachusetts

An Everything® Series Book.
Everything® and everything.com® are registered trademarks of F+W Publications, Inc.

Published by Adams Media, an F+W Publications Company
57 Littlefield Street, Avon, MA 02322 U.S.A.
www.adamsmedia.com

ISBN 10: 1-59869-245-3
ISBN 13: 978-1-59869-245-7

Printed in the United States of America.

J   I   H   G   F   E   D   C   B   A

Library of Congress Cataloging-in-Publication Data
Sember, Brette McWhorter.
The everything guide to pregnancy over 35 /
Brette McWhorter Sember, with Bruce D. Rodgers, and Diane E. Rodgers.
p. cm. — (An everything series book)
ISBN-13: 978-1-59869-245-7 (pbk.)
ISBN-10: 1-59869-245-3 (pbk.)
1. Pregnancy in middle age—Popular works. 2. Childbirth in
middle age—Popular works. I. Rodgers, Bruce D. II. Rodgers,
Diane E. III. Title. IV. Title: Everything guide to pregnancy
over thirty-five.
RG556.6.S46 2007
618.20084'4—dc22   2007015890

This publication is designed to provide accurate and authoritative information with regard to the subject matter covered. It is sold with the understanding that the publisher is not engaged in rendering legal, accounting, or other professional advice. If legal advice or other expert assistance is required, the services of a competent professional person should be sought.

—From a *Declaration of Principles* jointly adopted by a Committee of the American Bar Association and a Committee of Publishers and Associations

Many of the designations used by manufacturers and sellers to distinguish their products are claimed as trademarks. Where those designations appear in this book and Adams Media was aware of a trademark claim, the designations have been printed with initial capital letters.

This book is available at quantity discounts for bulk purchases.
For information, please call 1-800-289-0963.

Contents

Top Ten Reasons to
Have a Baby after Age 35

1. Age is just a number. Motherhood always gives you a young soul.

2. Having a baby after 35 is not risky and is likely to go smoothly.

3. You've reached a point in your life where you have almost everything else you want. Now it's time to share it with a baby.

4. Being married or partnered is wonderful, but being parents is truly fantastic.

5. It's never too late to give your child a sibling.

6. Mr. Right hasn't shown up and there's no reason to wait any longer to be a mom.

7. You *can* do it all.

8. Creating a child is your contribution to the future.

9. There are more options than ever before on the pathway to motherhood. All you have to do is choose one.

10. You will never regret the decision to become a mother, but you might regret deciding to skip it.

Introduction

▶ A LOT IS MADE of "older" women getting pregnant and having babies. Women start worrying about their biological clock ticking even in their twenties and women over 35 are trained to think that they can't have a normal pregnancy. However, today's over-35 woman has an excellent chance of conceiving, having a healthy pregnancy, and delivering a perfect baby.

More and more women are starting or adding to their families after age 35, so much so that this threshold has become less of a serious concern for doctors and has instead simply become one of the many pieces of a medical history that a woman brings with her to pregnancy.

An over-35 pregnancy is not constantly under the microscope. Your health-care provider will probably tell you that you will most likely have a boring, regular pregnancy, with the exciting result of a beautiful baby. While there are things the over-35 woman needs to be educated and aware of, this does not mean you need to be worried or nervous. Your body can handle the work of creating a baby on its own. In the meantime, there are many decisions you can focus on, such as child care, arranging your career to accommodate a baby, preparing financially, and ways to commemorate your pregnancy.

The Everything® Guide to Pregnancy Over 35 is designed to answer your questions and concerns about all of the issues and concern that may accompany an over-35 pregnancy. This book is also your guide to the lifestyle changes your pregnancy may bring, which are significantly different than those that younger women may face. Whether this is your first baby or an addition to your family, pregnancy is a time of great change. Not only are you growing a person inside you (how amazing is that?), you're also finding a way to adjust your career, relationship, home, responsibilities, and activities to accommodate the changes to your body and the changes that will soon be happening to your life.

Your pregnancy should be a partnership with your trusted health-care provider, but when it comes to the bottom line, it's your body, and you are the one who needs to be informed and make decisions. This book will help you do that with the confidence that your pregnancy will be a happy and wonderful time for you and your baby.

Chapter 1

Deciding to Become a Parent

Deciding to become a parent is one of the most significant decisions you can make in your life. For some women, it is something they have always known they wanted. For others, it is something they realize over time. Thinking about this decision can be emotional, and it can be even more complicated when you are over age 35. Do you really want to be a mother? Can you get pregnant? Can you have a healthy baby? These are all questions many women over 35 confront, work through, and find the answers to as well.

Evaluating If You Want a Child

Choosing to have a child is a complicated decision, one women have been dealing with ever since they were able to control their fertility. Not all women are meant to be or want to become mothers. Sometimes it may seem that society simply expects you to have a child. You've probably dealt with relatives and friends asking when and if you'll have children. By the time you reach age 35, the questioning can get a bit old!

Deciding whether or you not want to become a mother is a personal decision and one that you must make on your own or with your partner, if you have one. What's right for other women may not be right for you, and you must make a choice that will help you shape your life the way you want it.

Tick, Tock

When you are over age 35, you may feel pressured to make a decision and make it quickly. After all, you think, that biological clock is steadily moving forward. However, this is a decision that can't be rushed and must be made in its own time. You need to look at your life as a whole and evaluate what you really want, what will truly make you happy, and what elements of your life are non-negotiable. While it is true that women have a limited window of fertility, it is also true that women are having children at later stages of life now more than ever. The last thing you want to do is rush into something without examining your true desires.

What to Consider

Having a baby is a momentous occurrence that will influence every single area of your life. It is truly a life-changing event, one that most women who choose to follow that path find changes things for the better. Becoming a mother alters who you are forever and reconfigures your life permanently. Sound scary? It is a bit, but becoming a mother also changes your life in such a way that you simply can't and wouldn't want to imagine life without your child.

At this stage in your life, though, this is a choice that you want to think through completely.

As a parent, you will experience changes in all aspects of your life, including these:

- Finances
- Career
- Living arrangement/housing
- Free time
- Friendships
- Family relationships
- Long-term goals and plans
- Energy
- Emotions
- Health

You need to weigh the considerable impact a child will have on these areas of your life and decide if these changes are ones you want to have in your life. It's okay if you decide that you don't want to live a life with the changes a child will bring; many women make that same choice and live a happy and completely fulfilled life. You must make a decision that is right for you.

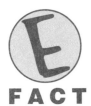

Child-free living is a growing trend. According to the National Center for Health Statistics, in 1975, about one in eleven women were living a child-free life by the age of 44. But by 1993, that number had risen to approximately one in six. At that time, 34.9 million American families were child free, and only 33.3 million families had a child under the age of 18.

Your Various Options

If you think you are interested in having a child, you have many, many options available to you. You can have a baby the traditional way, through a pregnancy with your partner. Traditional pregnancy doesn't work out for everyone, and you may decide you don't want to follow that route. There are other options available to you if you reach one of these conclusions. You can also adopt a baby, use insemination, use an egg donor, use a surrogate, or adopt an older child.

If you love children and want them to be a part of your life, there are other options and considerations. One choice is to become a foster parent. Foster parents provide loving homes for children who are removed from their parents' homes due to abuse or neglect. Foster parents care for the children until they are returned to their parents or until they are freed for adoption.

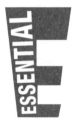

Learn more about foster parenting through the Dave Thomas Foundation for Adoption, online at *www.davethomasfoundationforadoption.org* or by phone at 800-275-3832. Get more information about Big Brothers/ Big Sisters of America at their Web site *www.bbbs.org* and use their locator to find your local agency.

There are also Big Brother/Big Sister programs that pair adults with kids who need guidance and friendship. Many schools have mentoring programs where adults help kids read, assist with homework, teach the basics of business, or just provide support. You might also consider a career change so that you could become a teacher and work with children every day.

Making Room in Your Life for a Child

If you decide that you do want to bring a child into your life, you already realize that you'll have to make some changes. Pregnancy brings many physical changes that immediately impact your life. Caring for a baby, toddler, preschooler, and child of any age brings its own challenges, rewards, and needs. You will always be changing and growing with your child throughout the years to come.

Here is a small snapshot of some of the changes you might find yourself making as you raise a child:

- **Pregnancy:** You may find yourself to be extremely tired at times and unable to do some of things you enjoy, like jogging or rock climbing. You'll surrender to the physical changes and buy a new wardrobe. Alcohol, cigarettes, certain fish and cheeses, and many medications will be off limits.

- **Newborn:** As you work to get your body back, you may find that it won't be entirely yours for quite a long time as you nurse, get up for nighttime feedings, and feel completely physically attached to your baby. Leaving her may be difficult, and you'll find that your living space explodes into a complete baby world.

- **Older baby:** You'll be shocked at how quickly your little one outgrows each size. You'll need a sitter if you want to head out to a movie. If you're back to work, planning for day care alone is not enough. You'll also need backup day care in case baby gets sick.

- **Toddler:** The days of spending an afternoon at the mall are long gone, since naptime cuts into the day. If you thought you were tired carrying a baby around, you'll soon find that toddlers require just as much energy and even more patience. Mealtimes can be complicated with picky eaters.

- **Preschool:** Play dates are a big part of your life and by now you know the theme songs to many children's television shows by heart. Your living area is probably overflowing with toys made up of many little pieces. Staying out late with your little one isn't an option since any bedtime later than 8 p.m. throws everything out of whack.

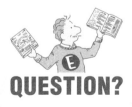

QUESTION?

What are the Mommy Wars?
The Mommy Wars are a difference of opinion among some women about the best way to raise children. Some mothers firmly believe that it is wrong for mothers to work and that all mothers should stay home with their children. Other mothers firmly believe that working while mothering is the best option. There is no right answer; each woman must make a decision about what is best for her and her family.

Impact on Your Career

Having a baby can completely turn your career on its head, or it can have little impact. There are mothers who have experienced it both ways. The effect a baby will have on your job is really something only you can determine. It is possible to continue at your job, working the same hours, on the same path to success as you were on before becoming a parent. However, many women find that because of the physical and emotional needs of a baby, it can be difficult to continue to work.

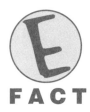

Fewer mothers are choosing to work while raising their children. In 2003, the U.S. Census Bureau reported there were 5.4 million stay-at-home moms in the United States. This followed their 2002 report, which found that only 55 percent of mothers with infant children worked, down from a record 59 percent in 1998. This is the first significant decline since the Census Bureau began tracking this number in 1976.

When you are considering whether or not to have a baby, you need to think about how important your career is to you. Your job probably has a lot of importance in your life. You may financially need the income you earn. Doing your job well probably makes you feel accomplished and satisfied. You may have established a circle of friends and colleagues who are important in your life. And as it is for many women, your job may be a large part of your identity. All of these factors are things to consider when you think about the impact a child may have on your career.

Stay-at-Home Parenting

Many women choose to stay at home with their babies. Leaving your job and staying at home means you will lose the income your job provides, but you may also find you have a reduction in expenses. You may be able to cut the following items from your budget:

- Work clothes
- Commuting costs
- Food and beverages at work
- Work-related gifts
- Organizational items like briefcase, calendar, and BlackBerry

Additionally, you would not have to factor in the cost of child care, which you would bear if you did continue to work.

Choosing to stay-at-home with your baby does not have to be a life sentence. Being a stay-at-home mom is a wonderful, fulfilling choice for many women. You have the opportunity to witness every milestone and be the primary caregiver for your child. You also have the ability to spend time with your other children, if you have any, and take the time to run your household in a very hands-on way. At-home moms do an important job and for many women it is a time in their lives they wouldn't trade for anything. Many women leave their jobs and later return to their careers when their children are older. It can be difficult to re-enter the workforce after years away, but it is becoming a more common option that works for many moms.

Working and Parenting

Millions of women work while caring for their children, and choosing to do so does not mean you are a bad mother or selfish person. If your job is essential to your family finances, something that gives you self-esteem and a sense of well being, or is just simply something that you want to keep doing, you should be applauded for making a decision that works for your family. Mothering and working is a juggling act no matter how you look at it, but it can be a wonderfully fulfilling life. Moms who work have the best of both worlds: a satisfying career and home life.

When deciding if you want to return to your job after your child joins your family, consider the following:

- **Child care:** Child care will be a major concern for your family. You will need to make a plan that you feel most comfortable with and that best accommodates your needs.
- **Breastfeeding:** If you want to nurse your baby, you will need to make arrangements to pump while you are away from your baby.

There are terrific pumps available, and most employers are willing to make accommodations for nursing moms.

- **Scheduling:** As a working mom, you might find that you can no longer be quite as flexible at work; you may need to leave at a set time each day to pick up your child from the child-care provider.
- **Family time:** Spending time with your baby and family is likely to be a priority to you, and this may make it difficult to bring work home, go on business trips, or work on weekends.
- **Mental energy:** Doing your job successfully while also parenting can be draining, physically and mentally. Working moms have to find a way to divvy up their energy and focus.
- **Guilt:** Unfortunately, many working moms deal with guilt. When they're at work, they feel guilty for not spending time with their children. When they're with their children, they feel guilty for not focusing on work. It can become a difficult cycle.

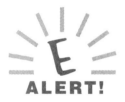

ALERT!

All mothers feel guilt. No matter how well you plan your life, weigh the options, and make rational choices, odds are that you'll feel guilty some of the time. It can't be avoided. All you can do is live your life to the best of your ability. Enjoy the joyful moments that motherhood brings and try not to let yourself get bogged down by any perceived negatives.

Other Options

You aren't limited to the two options of being a stay-at-home mom or working full time. There is a whole array of other possibilities. Many women take time off under their employer's maternity leave plan or through the Family and Medical Leave Act to be with their baby for several months and then return to work. Working part-time appeals to many women and allows you to have some income while still spending a lot of time at home. Flex-time, where you work the same number of hours but at irregular times (such as working four ten-hour days instead of five eight-hour days) and job-sharing (in which you and another employee do one full-time job together) are other choices. Some women do freelance or consulting work from home, while others choose to be involved in charity or school organizations. Your partner also has the same options for his or her job, and parenting is a job that definitely encourages cooperation.

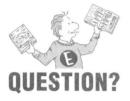

QUESTION?

What is the Family and Medical Leave Act?

The Family and Medical Leave Act (FMLA) is a federal law that requires employers with more than fifty employees to allow parents to take up to twelve weeks of unpaid leave in a twelve-month period to care for a newborn or newly adopted child. This is an option available to employees who have worked for the same employer for over one year. Both moms and dads can take time off under this law.

Impact on Your Relationships

Having a baby often results in a reordering of priorities, including your relationships. Babies are time-intensive, and many women find that they have less time for friends, relatives, and even their partner after a baby enters their lives. As a new mom, your baby takes priority, particularly when you are adjusting to the newness of the situation. And when you're not with your baby, you may feel quite tired and prefer a few hours of sleep to spending time with a friend.

Friends

As important as your friends are, they can end up taking a back seat to parenthood. Many women find that their friendships shift after having children. Friends who have children simply understand and relate better than childless friends. There is less time to hang out with friends and do adult activities. This does not mean that women who have children lose all their childless friends; however, you may find that it takes a little more effort to maintain your friendships after your little one arrives.

Relatives

Family members often become closer after the birth of a child. Everyone wants to see the new baby, and the baby's grandparents, aunts, and uncles often clamor for the right to baby-sit and visit. Seeing that much of your family might be quite a change, but often a baby brings you closer to your female relatives, who now can relate to you on a completely new level.

Your Partner

Becoming parents is a whole new stage of your committed relationship and is a wonderful new way to rediscover each other. However, as glorious as it might be to see your partner become a parent, the stress and sleep deprivation of new parenthood can magnify existing problems in your relationship. Suddenly a toilet seat left up can become the end of the world. And the hormones associated with pregnancy and the postpartum period can certainly make things quite difficult.

Parenting together requires a new kind of cooperation, understanding, and skill. You'll likely see new and amazing things in your partner as you simultaneously become outraged at his or her inability to fasten snaps on baby clothes. Deciding to become parents together is something that can never be undone. For the rest of your lives, you will be that child's parents together no matter what. It is an awesome undertaking and a giant commitment to each other and to your child.

Impact on Your Finances

Having a baby drains your bank account, yet it pays you back in immeasurable love. Babies are not cheap. Many people think they are, for how can something so small that only drinks free breast milk be expensive? Babies are in fact a huge expense.

The costs begin in pregnancy, when you have regular medical expenses, the cost of classes and books, and an entire new wardrobe for yourself. Move on to birth, with hospital costs for mom and baby. Then consider loss of income from taking time off or leaving or cutting back your hours at work, or from your partner doing the same thing. If one of you needs to switch to a family health insurance policy, there may be additional costs there. Then consider the costs of diapers, baby clothes, baby equipment, baby toys and books, baby food, formula, baby doctor visits, child care, and more. If you need a bigger home at some point, you'll have the costs of that as well. In short, babies are not cheap, and they don't get any less expensive as they grow older.

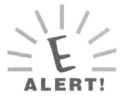

ALERT!

It costs the average family approximately $269,000 to raise a child from birth to age seventeen, according to the U.S. Department of Agriculture. And that does not take into account the cost of college! All told, that tiny little bundle of joy will end up costing you well over a third of a million dollars.

Benefits of Being a Mom Over 35

It may seem as though all you hear about these days are the risks of being an older mom. While there are some medical differences in pregnancy for older moms (discussed in detail in later chapters), there are many benefits to being an older mom that you might not hear people discuss often.

Being an older mom means you are in fact more experienced. This means you're more likely to be able to handle the pressures and challenges of parenthood with more patience and wisdom than a younger woman. You know who you are and have had time to sow your wild oats, explore your world, and try different things. You're likely quite ready to settle down and be a mom for a while.

Older mothers tend to be more financially stable than younger mothers, and their partners are also usually more financially prepared to be a parent. Older moms are more likely to have stable careers and have partners with stable careers. (Stable careers mean stable income.) Older mothers also are more likely to have a better understanding of how to manage money and tend to have larger nest eggs built up. As a woman who has probably worked for many years, it is likely you are at a good point in your career, and taking time off to have a baby isn't as detrimental to you as it could be to a younger, less-established woman.

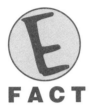

FACT

According to the U.S. Census Bureau, the average age at which a U.S. woman gives birth for the first time is now 25.1 years. That may seem young to you, but in 1970 it was 21.1 years! Approximately 5 percent of all births in the United States are to women over age 35.

If you've been wanting a baby for a long time, have been trying to get pregnant for a long time, or have used reproductive technology to help you conceive, you're probably very pleased and relieved to be pregnant. Because of this, it's likely you'll better be able to view the whole pregnancy and parenting experience with perspective. It's likely that you have a good support system in place as well, and that you have sisters, friends, sisters-in-law, cousins, and so on who have children and can give you advice and offer a helping hand when you need one.

Chapter 2

Avenues to Parenthood

Beyond the traditional male-and-female married couple conceiving a baby, there are a wide variety of ways to become a parent. Today there are many choices for women who want to become parents. To be a parent you don't have to be married, heterosexual, or even become pregnant. Families are built on love, not on technicalities. Additionally, many women become parents after miscarriages or without planning. However you get there, the journey is just as wonderful and the result is the same—a child to love.

Single Moms

You don't need a husband to have a baby, and many women are going ahead and realizing their dreams of being mothers without being married to a man. If you choose to have a child on your own, you certainly won't be alone. Because so many divorced mothers raise children alone, single mothers are considered nothing out of the ordinary.

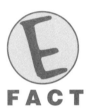

FACT

According to the U.S. Census Bureau, more than a third of all babies (34.6 percent, to be exact) are born to single, unmarried moms. For support and information, join Single Mothers by Choice (*http://mattes .home.pipeline.com*; 212-988-0993) or the National Organization of Single Mothers (*www.singlemothers.org*; 704-888-5437).

Raising a child by yourself is certainly a doable proposition. While it's true you won't have a partner there to help you with colic, diaper duty, or midnight feedings, it also means that you'll be your child's favorite person. Parenting alone is manageable if you have a good support system in place that is made up of family, friends, child-care professionals, and medical professionals. There are several pathways to single motherhood to consider.

Known Father

Perhaps the simplest way to become a single mother is to become pregnant from intercourse with a man in your life. The best course of action is to talk to the man you have in mind and agree that you want to create a child together.

If the man you would like to be the father doesn't want to be a real involved father to your child, you can either simply put "unknown" on the birth certificate for father, or you can see an attorney and have formal papers drawn up that give you complete custody and relieve him of any responsibility for child support. When thinking about single motherhood, many women consider how they will find male role models for their child and how their extended family will react to the decision to parent alone.

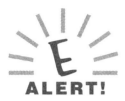

ALERT!

Remember that any man who is the biological father of a child is entitled to seek custody or visitation. Even if you and a man in your life agree to create a child without him involved as a parent, he can always change his mind and go to court. Having an attorney draw up a legal, binding custody agreement is important no matter how much you are in agreement.

Sperm Donor

Another option is to use a sperm donor to help you create a child. You can obtain a donation from a man you know or have a relationship with. (This is different from just having a baby together; sperm donors sign legal documents prior to the donation giving up all rights to the child.) Once you've reached an agreement, you can create a child the natural way or through insemination.

Sperm banks are another option. Sperm banks pay donors to donate sperm. Donor sperm is carefully screened for STDs and medical conditions. The sperm is frozen until testing is complete (HIV testing takes several months to complete). The women receiving the donations also must be tested for STDs. Donors are described in a data bank or often in a booklet. Information available about the donor often includes the following:

- Photos of the donor as an adult and/or as a child
- Complete medical history
- Physical attributes
- Mental abilities
- Occupation
- Hobbies
- Personality traits
- Nationality

Some women have specific traits in mind when looking for a donor, and when you use a sperm bank you can be very particular.

The sperm bank provides counseling to the donors and the women who receive the donations. There is a fee (between $200 and $400) for purchasing the sperm. You can find a list of sperm banks at *www.fertilityplus.org/faq/donor.html*. Once you have chosen a donor, you can either choose to do a home insemination yourself or have your physician perform a medical insemination. Medical insemination involves a catheter being inserted into the cervical opening (intracervical insemination) or through the cervix so the sperm can be deposited directly in the uterus (intrauterine insemination), increasing the odds of a pregnancy occurring. The latter method is often done in infertility treatment because of male infertility factors. Intrauterine insemination requires the sperm to be washed so as to remove chemicals from the semen that may cause serious reactions. The American Society of Reproductive Medicine provides a booklet about insemination on their Web site at *www.asrm.org/Literature/patient.html*.

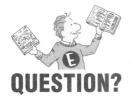

QUESTION?

How do I choose a sperm bank?
There is currently no federal regulation of sperm banks in the United States. Because of this, it is important to find a sperm bank that is accredited by the American Association of Tissue Banks (*www.aatb.org*) and which follows the guidelines recommended by the American Society of Reproductive Medicine (ASRM) (*www.asrm.org*).

When you use a sperm donor, you receive a complete medical history for the donor. Some sperm banks have mechanisms in place so that children of donors are notified of medical conditions discovered in the donor or donor's family years after the donation takes place. Some donors are willing to be contacted by their children in the future, while others wish not to be. If this is an important consideration for you, discuss it with the sperm bank. You may also wish to ask to have several other vials of the same donor's sperm reserved for you in case you would like to have more children, so that they can be full siblings to each other. It's important to ask how many children a donor you are considering has. If there are many, you may wish to consider using another donor, because this increases the odds that his children could someday meet and could unwittingly have children together.

Adoption

Adoption is a pathway to parenthood that works for both single and married women. Adoption allows you to give the gift of a family to a child who might not otherwise have one. When you adopt a child, he legally becomes your child, and a new birth certificate is issued with your name as parent. Some women worry that adopting a child is not the same as having a biological child. Women who have adopted can tell you that you will love an adoptive child just as much as any other child in your family and biology doesn't make a bit of difference. Once that child is placed in your arms, she becomes yours. Adoption is simply another pathway to finding the child of your heart.

All adoptions require the adoptive parents to obtain a home study and criminal background check to be eligible to adopt. A home study is a written document prepared by a social worker that describes your situation, including the following:

- Job and work commitments
- Finances
- Marital status
- Living arrangements
- Child-care arrangements you would make
- Physical and mental health
- Support system, including family and friends
- Hobbies and interests

In addition to the home study document and various court forms, you'll be asked to provide several letters of recommendation from people in your life, such as clergy, friends, and neighbors. It can seem a little exhausting that you have to prove yourself to such an extent when other women can get pregnant without any approval from anyone, but the system is set up to protect children.

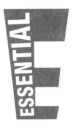

An open adoption is one in which the birth parents and adoptive parents have some contact with each other. In a closed adoption, information about the birth parents is kept private. Many people also think of an open adoption as being one in which the child is told about his or her birth parents.

All adoptions must be finalized with a court proceeding, and you should always use an attorney. Contact the American Academy of Adoption Attorneys for a referral (*www.adoptionattorneys.org*; 202-832-2222).

When considering adoption, there are several types to choose from, including international, domestic public agency, domestic private agency, and independent adoption.

International Adoption

International adoption is the adoption of a child from a country outside the United States. The benefit of international adoption is that there are many children available. Because of the waiting periods, these children cannot be adopted as newborns.

The cost of an international adoption is somewhere between $10,000 and $40,000, about the same as a domestic adoption once you add in travel costs. (With most international adoptions, you must travel to your child's country of origin at least once.) When you do an international adoption, you almost always need to work through a U.S. agency that works with an agency in the foreign country. In some countries you are able to choose your child yourself, while other countries simply assign a child to you. There are often unplanned holdups and red tape involved in international adoptions, so it is important to work with an agency that will support you entirely and work through these snags with you. You'll want to be sure the agency provides you with an interpreter and a representative to help move things along while you are traveling.

It is essential that you retain an attorney who is experienced in handling international adoptions because completing the process is all about having the paperwork done correctly. To have the adoption recognized by the

U.S. government, you will probably need to adopt your child in the country of origin and then repeat the procedure at home in your state. You will also need to complete immigration paperwork prior to bringing your child home, to obtain permission to bring him into the country.

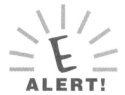

ALERT!

When planning an international adoption, it is important that you find a pediatrician who specializes in international adoption so that he or she can evaluate the photos and medical records you receive of potential adoptive children. This allows you to make an informed choice about whether you want to adopt the child in question, who may have medical conditions common in certain developing countries.

When you do an international adoption, you often do not meet or receive any information about your child's birth parents and may not have any way of finding them when your child is older. However, many parents find that international adoption brings a whole new culture into their lives and allows them to explore their child's culture and incorporate it into the family. It is possible to raise your child as an American while celebrating and embracing his heritage.

Domestic Public Agency Adoption

A public adoption agency is one run by a state, and the children available for adoption are by and large children who were placed in foster care and have now been freed for adoption. The biological parents of these children had their parental rights terminated, and the children are placed in foster care until an adoptive family can be found for them. Many of these children are older and because of this, they can be hard to place. Additionally there are often sibling groups of children that need to be placed together, something few families are willing to do. The benefit of state agency adoption is that there is no shortage of children available; however, it is next to impossible to adopt a newborn this way. Public agency adoptions are the least expensive type of adoption, with costs averaging about $3,000.

You may be able to accept a child as a legal risk placement, which entails having him placed in your home before the adoption is officially completed so that you can immediately begin bonding with each other. Many public agency adoptive children have special needs, so it is important to obtain a full assessment and discuss financial assistance available for these children. You will also want to know about the child's exposure to, or use of, drugs or alcohol.

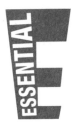

To find children available for adoption through state agencies, view their photos online through the state photo listings at *http://photolisting.adoption.com*. You can also contact your local department of social services or family and children's services for information about children in your area.

Another consideration in public agency adoption is that many of these children know who their biological parents are. An adoption may sever all legal ties to the biological parents, but it can't erase memories or change a child's attachment to a parent. Because of this, many courts allow adoptive and biological parents to create kinship agreements—written agreements that allow the child to continue to have contact with biological parents, siblings, and other relatives. These agreements are not usually legally binding, though, and are at the discretion of the adoptive parents.

Domestic Private Agency Adoption

Adoption through a private U.S. agency is what most people think of when they hear the word *adoption*. This is the type of adoption through which you are able to adopt newborns, but there may be long waits, with some lasting over a year. In a domestic private agency adoption, you must first choose an agency to work with. Attend several informational meetings and choose an agency that you feel most comfortable with. Ask for references and check them.

A private agency adoption can cost up to $40,000. Get details about how the fee is broken down and what part is refundable if an adoption does not occur. The adoptive parents pay the birth mother's medical expenses. Be sure to inquire if you will be paying your birth mother's personal medical expenses or whether you will pay into a pool that covers expenses for all birth mothers. The pool is a gamble given that your birth mother's expenses could be higher or lower than the average.

Birth mothers contact agencies about placing their babies. Birth parents are then screened by the agency, which chooses only those who are sincere. The agency then selects an adoptive parent or parents, or the birth mother may make the selection. The agency handles all contact with the birth mother unless the parties agree to have personal contact. Counseling is required. You usually will meet the birth mother at least once (more if you have an open adoption arrangement), and you will have a complete medical history for your child.

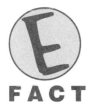

FACT

In 1992, the last year for which adoption statistics have been gathered, the National Center for State Courts reported that 126,951 children were adopted in the United States. Over 1.5 million U.S. children have been adopted, 2 percent of all children.

In most states there is a waiting period (ranging from a few days to a few weeks) between the birth and when the birth parent's rights are formally revoked. This is the time period in which birth parents can change their minds, and this is what most adoptive parents worry about the most when considering adoption. The good news is that birth parents rarely change their minds. In the cases that get media attention, it is usually true that both the birth parents did not give legal and binding consent to the adoption.

Independent Adoption

An independent adoption occurs when you locate a birth mother yourself without the help of an agency. There are several ways to locate a birth mother. A popular way is to place ads in the newspaper, asking potential birth mothers to contact you. You can use word of mouth, asking people to spread the word. Some adoptive parents have business cards made up with their contact information so that can be passed along. Creating a Web site about yourself is another way to get the word out about your desire to adopt.

There are many Web sites where you can register and place ads or notices. Another method is to work with an adoption attorney who has information about birth mothers seeking adoptive parents. Yet another method is to use an adoption facilitator, a professional who works to put birth parents in touch with adoptive parents.

The benefit of independent adoption is that you alone are in control. No agency makes decisions about you. You find a birth mother, and you decide if she is right for you. You also can adopt a newborn and create whatever kind of open adoption arrangement works for all involved.

As with private agency adoption, you always run the risk that the birth parents will change their minds. If you're on your own, you have no backup and no agency to find another baby for you right away. There are very specific laws about adoption governing everything from the types of ads you can place to the way contact is initiated to what expenses you are allowed to pay for. It is essential that you work with an experienced attorney who can guide you through the process.

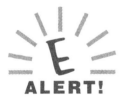

ALERT!

Adoption facilitators are specifically permitted by law in only four states. Twenty-three states prohibit them. Other states have no laws either way. Because facilitators are not very well accepted, if you choose to use one, be certain to get references and have an attorney review all documents.

It is very important that you and the birth mother each see a counselor to help you deal with the emotions associated with adoption. It is a very difficult decision for the birth mother to make, and you want to be sure she is committed to it before you invest time and money.

It is possible to find a birth mother on your own and then hire an agency to see the adoption through. With this method, you make the important choice of birth mother yourself and then obtain professional help with the details of the adoption.

Blended Families

A wonderful way to have a parenting relationship with a child is to be a stepparent. If you are married to or plan to marry someone who has children from a previous relationship, you are or will be a stepparent to them. The relationship is sometimes portrayed as difficult, but if you keep in mind that your stepchildren have two parents and have the bonus of having another adult in their lives who loves them, you will be able to keep it all in perspective.

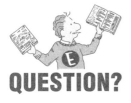

QUESTION?

What legal rights do stepparents have with regard to their stepchildren?

Stepparents have few legal rights to their stepchildren. Stepparents are not legal parents unless they formally adopt their stepchildren. (Called a second-parent adoption, this is a shorter, simpler process than other adoptions.) Some courts have begun recognizing the emotional bond that exists between stepparents and stepchildren, but they are not the majority.

Should you have a child of your own, your children and your spouse's children will be stepsiblings. Blended families such as these are more and more common today, when so many marriages end in divorce. Raising a blended family requires patience, schedules, and good communication.

Same-Sex Couples

If you have a same-sex partner, it is very possible to become parents together. In most states, one of you will have to become a parent first. The other parent then adopts the child through the second-parent adoption process used by stepparents. A second-parent adoption is a simplified adoption, but it does still require a home study and background checks.

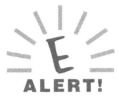

ALERT!

A second-parent adoption is absolutely essential if you and your partner are raising a child together. Should the legal parent die, the partner has no legal ties to the child and may not be given custody, even if a will names her as guardian. A second-parent adoption ensures that both of you are legal parents.

Many lesbian couples choose to use insemination to become pregnant. As discussed earlier in the chapter, you can use a known donor or go to a sperm bank. Some lesbian couples prefer to use sperm donations from gay donors. If this is something you are interested in, there is a sperm bank in San Francisco called Rainbow Flag Health Services (*www.gayspermbank.com*) that specializes in these kinds of donations.

Adoption is another choice for same-sex couples. If you are considering international adoption, you should be aware that no foreign countries permit gay couples to adopt. Homosexuality has become a "Don't ask, don't tell" situation in the adoption community to some extent. If you are gay and you are adopting a child alone, with plans for your partner to do a second-parent adoption later, there is no need to disclose this. When you have a home study done, you will have to be honest about living with someone else, but it is possible to paint this as a roommate situation.

Some private domestic agencies are funded by churches and may have preferences against gay couples. Public agencies are most likely to be accepting to gay singles or couples.

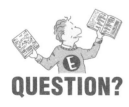

QUESTION?

How do I find a lesbian-friendly sperm bank?
Most sperm banks are now very lesbian-friendly and don't care if a woman is married, single, or gay. For a list of sperm banks that are known to be lesbian-friendly, visit *www.familypride.org* and read the FAQs in the education section.

If one of you has a child from a previous relationship, the other partner can adopt the child. If the child has a second legal parent, that parent must receive notice of and consent to the adoption. If the other parent will not consent, then your partner won't be able to formally adopt your child.

Unplanned Pregnancy

If you are pregnant and did not plan the pregnancy, you're probably still in shock. Unplanned pregnancies can cause a whole host of emotions—fear, joy, anger, sadness, excitement, anxiety, and more. It can take time to adjust to the idea of becoming a mother, and a mature mother at that.

If you talk to parents of other unplanned children, though, you will find that they would not change the fact of their child's existence for the world. Take some time and talk with your partner, family, and friends if you are feeling a little shaky at the idea of being a mother. The most important thing you can do is see your obstetrician or midwife as soon as possible and begin taking a prenatal vitamin immediately. Try to pinpoint the first day of your last period so that your health-care provider can determine how far along you are. You will probably be offered an ultrasound to accurately date the pregnancy.

Pregnancy after Loss

Many women experience pregnancy loss and go on to have other children. The miscarriage rate is difficult to pinpoint because many miscarriages occur before the woman realizes she is pregnant. With current technology, a pregnancy can be (but often is not) diagnosed as early as nine days after conception, even before a period is missed. Including these early confirmed pregnancies, as many as 20 to 50 percent of all pregnancies end in miscarriage. About 15 percent of all clinically confirmed (by fetal heart rate or ultrasound) pregnancies end in miscarriage.

When you get pregnant again after a pregnancy loss, you are likely to be very worried about experiencing another loss. Some women feel extremely nervous until they pass the point at which the previous pregnancy ended. Try to take things one day at a time and avoid worrying unnecessarily. Talk to your physician about your concerns and discuss any risk factors. The majority of miscarriages are chromosomally abnormal or have embryos with serious birth defects; in most cases, it is the mother's body's way of dealing with an abnormal pregnancy. Generally, having one miscarriage does not increase the risk of a second miscarriage. For the most part, you are likely to have a happy and healthy pregnancy this time around. The loss that you suffered will never completely leave you, and you may still find yourself noticing the due date for that pregnancy go by or other milestones. The child that you lost will always be a part of you.

Facing Pregnancy Again

If you have other children and are pregnant again, you may be thrilled and excited or you may be apprehensive. If this is your first over-35 pregnancy, you may be wondering how it will be different from your previous pregnancies. Your obstetrician or midwife may monitor your pregnancy a bit more closely; you might find you tire a bit more easily than with previous pregnancies; and you may have more prenatal testing to get through. But if you've been pregnant before, you can rest assured that this pregnancy will probably be similar to your previous pregnancy or pregnancies.

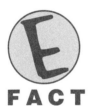

FACT

According to the U.S. Census Bureau, the average U.S. family has 1.86 children. The state with the highest average is Utah, where families average 2.21 children. Your family certainly won't have any decimal points!

If you already have children, you are probably excited about adding a sibling to your family. You'll now be dividing your energies between your existing child or children and your pregnancy and soon-to-be newborn. Adding a child to your family means learning some juggling skills and managing sibling conflicts, but it also means having the joy of watching your children love each other. You will find the right balance in your life and your new family will fit into your life.

Chapter 3

Fertility

One of the greatest worries you may be facing is whether it is too late for you to get pregnant or if you will have difficulty getting pregnant because of your age. The good news is that most women over 35 who want to have babies will successfully do so. Even if you experience some difficulty, there are so many options and treatments available that you will have many opportunities to consider and try.

Your Biological Clock

Although a woman's fertility does start to decline after age 35, becoming pregnant is still a very viable possibility. The decline in fertility is a gradual one. There is not a sudden drop-off, where you're as fertile as the proverbial rabbit at age 34 and suddenly barren at age 35. Your body changes gradually over years. The average age for menopause is 51, so there are still many years left for childbearing, whether you are in your 30s or 40s.

According to the Mayo Clinic, female fertility peaks between age 20 and 24. From age 30 to 35, fertility is 15 to 20 percent below maximum. From age 35 to 39, it's down 25 to 50 percent, and from age 40 to 45, the decrease is 50 to 95 percent. There are several reasons why fertility can decline after age 35, including fibroids, ovulation problems, and endometriosis.

Endometriosis

Endometriosis is a condition in which the tissue that normally grows inside the uterus (the endometrium) grows outside the uterus. It attaches to the ovaries or fallopian tubes and elsewhere in the abdomen and makes it difficult for an egg to be released or travel through the tubes. When a woman gets her period, the endometrium creates the blood that is released. Women with endometriosis bleed from all their endometrial tissue, and this can become trapped in the abdomen with no way to get out. Endometriosis is often a painful condition. It can be diagnosed by laparoscopy (surgery via small openings in the abdomen). Endometriosis becomes more common after age 35. While there is no ultimate cure, there are many treatment options, including surgery, hormone treatment, and pain medication.

Ovulation Problem

Achieving pregnancy is all about eggs and the quality of those eggs. As women age, the number and quality of eggs decrease. A woman is born with all the eggs she will ever have—no new ones are created. The eggs get used up throughout your life, and they also age and experience chromosomal problems. The number of eggs remaining is called the ovarian reserve, and it's something your doctor can test. These eggs are less likely to be released from the ovary (ovulation), implant successfully in the uterus, and are more likely to be chromosomally abnormal.

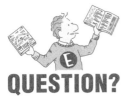

How likely am I to have trouble getting pregnant?
You actually have very good odds. A report in the medical journal *Contemporary OB/GYN* showed that about a third of women ages 35 to 39 had fertility problems. That number increased to 50 percent of women over age 40.

Many women (up to 10 percent) experience polycystic ovarian syndrome (PCOS), in which there is an imbalance of hormones and ovulation difficulties. Additionally, women over 40 are more likely to have an imbalance of male and female hormones, which can impact ovulation.

Fibroids

According to the American Institute for Preventive Medicine, 20 to 25 percent of women over 35 have fibroids (benign tumors that grow in the uterus). African American women, women with a family history of fibroids, and women who have not been pregnant are more likely to have them. Symptoms include heavy menstrual bleeding, pain, constipation, frequent urination, and anemia. Most fibroids are small and inconsequential. However, if they are large or impinge on the uterine lining and uterine cavity, it can be difficult for a fertilized egg to implant in the uterus.

Treatment involves surgical removal of the fibroids. Another treatment option is uterine artery embolization (UAE) or uterine fibroid embolization (UFE), in which a small catheter is inserted in the artery in the groin and threaded to the uterine arteries. Small particles are injected to block the blood supply to the fibroid, causing shrinkage. This is generally performed in women who are not contemplating pregnancy, but it has been performed in women who subsequently conceived and had normal pregnancies. It may be an option when the fibroid is so large that surgical removal itself may pose a risk of loss of the uterus.

Other Reasons

Another reason for declining fertility may include cervical mucous that is less hospitable to sperm. This is tested after coitus, generally one to two days within the time ovulation is expected. Several hours following intercourse, a sample of cervical mucous is obtained. The sample is examined to see that it "stretches" at least two inches, that it forms a "fern" pattern when drying, and that there are a normal number of live sperm actively swimming forward within it. The value of this test is somewhat disputed though it appears that a poor result indicates reduced fertility.

Uterine lining is another concern. The uterine lining is sampled to determine if the corpus luteum is functioning correctly. This forms within the ovary every month and makes progesterone to prepare the lining of the uterus for a pregnancy and to maintain the pregnancy through the first nine to ten weeks. If progesterone is not made sufficiently, infertility and/or early pregnancy loss can result. To test this, a uterine biopsy is done after ovulation to assess the effect of progesterone on the uterine lining. Generally, several tests must be performed to confirm the diagnosis, as every woman has occasional cycles in which the corpus luteum is insufficient. Treatment can include progesterone supplements during the luteal, or second, phase of the cycle or ovulation drugs to make ovulation stronger and the corpus luteum in that cycle more resilient. Some physicians prefer to do an ultrasound to evaluate the uterine lining.

Finding a Specialist

Most gynecologists are able to work with their patients to assist them on the pathway to conceiving a child. When you first decide you would like to have a baby, you need to go in for a preconception checkup. At this visit, you should discuss your age and health conditions with your doctor and specifically ask if you should see a specialist. The standard of care for women over age 35 is to try unassisted for six months and then begin fertility testing and treatment.

If your insurance will cover it, you have the right to seek out a specialist before this point. Should you decide to do so, or should your gynecologist recommend it, you will want to see a reproductive endocrinologist (RE) who is board certified. Reproductive endocrinologists are physicians who specialize in female fertility. Many reproductive endocrinologists practice in a group with urologists, labs, and facilities all in one place. It is important to realize that many gynecologists who are board certified in general obstetrics and gynecology will advertise themselves as "infertility specialists." These individuals should not be confused with reproductive endocrinologists (REs).

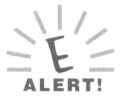

Many insurance plans do not cover fertility treatments. Only twelve states mandate some coverage for fertility treatments. Be sure to learn what your plan will cover before you undergo any treatments; an IVF cycle can cost over $10,000 alone. Some fertility clinics are able to arrange payment plans, so ask about them.

To find an RE, first ask for a referral from your gynecologist and check it against the list of participating physicians in your insurance plan. You should feel free to shop around until you find an RE you like. You may be able to get another referral from your family doctor. You can also use the find-a-physician feature of the American Society of Reproductive Medicine (at *www.asrm.org*).

Once you have the names of a few physicians that accept your insurance, make appointments with those you are considering. Use this appointment to ask questions and get a feel for the doctor's style. Questions to ask include these:

- How long have you been practicing this specialty?
- Are you board certified?
- Do you have a urologist on staff to evaluate male fertility?
- What is your office or clinic's rate of take-home babies?
- What kind of testing and treatment would you suggest for me?
- What kind of rate of success is involved?
- Based on my age, what do you think my odds might be?
- At what hospitals do you have privileges?

- What kind of financial arrangements can you make for treatments not covered by insurance?
- If I need advanced treatment, such as in-vitro fertilization, do you have the capabilities to perform these procedures, or will I have to be referred?

When you first see a specialist, she will meet with you and your partner and take a detailed medical history. You will be asked questions about not only your medical conditions but also about the frequency of intercourse and how many children you each have. Then the specialist will most likely order what is called a fertility workup, a series of tests (described later in this chapter) to assess the best course of treatment for you. An RE follows your care until you are pregnant and until a heartbeat is confirmed. At that point, you are turned back over to your OB/GYN or your maternal-fetal medicine specialist. (See Chapter 6 for more information.)

Determining If There Is a Problem

While most women are able to conceive on their own, if you and your partner have been trying for six months with no luck, it's time to see a doctor. Women under age 35 with good medical histories are advised to wait a year, but once you are over 35 and your fertility window is getting smaller, you should not wait any longer than six months. Women over age 40 shouldn't wait more than three months before seeking medical evaluation.

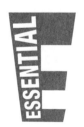

If you're having trouble getting pregnant, don't assume the problem is with your body. Male infertility is a contributing or sole factor in 40 percent of couples experiencing infertility problems, regardless of the age of the man or woman. Because of this, if you see a fertility specialist, it is essential that both of you be checked.

If you have been monitoring ovulation with a home ovulation test and basal body temperature (as described in Chapter 4) and as far as you can tell you are not ovulating, you should not wait six months. See your doctor as soon as possible. If you have irregular or unpredictable periods, you should not wait and should see your doctor. Additionally, if you have ever had pelvic inflammatory disease (PID) or an infection with chlamydia or gonorrhea, you should see your doctor. These infections can cause scarring of the fallopian tubes and make conception difficult.

Fertility Tests

There are a variety of fertility tests that can be done. A gynecologist can order some of these tests, but in general it makes sense to see a specialist who can order all necessary tests and treatments. These generally involve a medical evaluation, assessment of the uterine cavity and of the fallopian tubes, assessment of the male partner, and testing for ovulation. Additional tests may involve laparoscopy, assessment of cervical mucous, testing for polycystic ovarian syndrome, and in older women some test of ovarian reserve. In many cases no apparent cause will be found and the couple is said to have unexplained infertility. This does not mean that you cannot conceive; it just means that the cause of your infertility is not readily apparent. There are, in fact, many effective treatments for unexplained infertility.

Ovarian Reserve

Your doctor is able to test your body's number of viable eggs. This is done with a blood test on the second, third, or fourth day of your cycle. The blood test evaluates the levels of the hormones FSH and estradiol in your blood. High levels of the FSH hormone indicate low levels of ovarian reserve. Your physician may also have you take what is called the Clomid challenge test. You take the fertility drug Clomid, which stimulates ovulation, and then a blood test is done, measuring how well your body responded to the drug. Ovarian reserve can also be measured by ultrasound.

Progesterone Levels

Progesterone is the hormone that is released by a woman's body after ovulation and that helps prepare the uterus for implantation. Progesterone levels can be tested with a blood test after ovulation. Following ovulation, the area in the ovary from which ovulation occurred begins to produce progesterone, which prepares the uterine lining for the implantation of a fertilized egg.

Abnormal levels are known as luteal phase defect (LPD). Luteal phase defect may be suspected if your basal body temperature does not remain elevated for the usual twelve days after ovulation or if your menstrual cycles are short. Diagnosis is made by measuring post-ovulation progesterone levels or performing a timed endometrial biopsy.

Thyroid Levels

The thyroid is a gland in your neck that regulates hormone activity in your body. If your thyroid is not functioning properly, it can make it difficult to get pregnant. A simple blood test will check your level of TSH (thyroid stimulating hormone). If TSH levels are high it means you are thyroid deficient (hypothyroid), which can be corrected with thyroid replacement medication. This is important because there is evidence that even if the woman is only mildly hypothyroid, it can affect a baby's brain development.

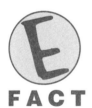

FACT

Infertility affects about 10 million Americans. According to the American Fertility Association, the probability of having a baby decreases 3 to 5 percent per year after the age of 30 and at a faster rate after 40.

If TSH levels are low, it means you are making too much thyroid hormone (hyperthyroid). There are options involving medication, radiation, or surgery to suppress the levels. The American Thyroid Association recommends that all people over age 35 get their thyroid levels checked at least once every five years. Any women contemplating pregnancy should have a preconception TSH test performed.

Pelvic Ultrasound

Pelvic ultrasound exams are used to check the condition of the uterus, tubes, and ovaries, and to track development of the follicle—the beginning stages of the egg. A woman will be asked to come in for several ultrasounds at the beginning of her cycle. These ultrasounds are usually done with a probe in the vagina and are not painful. The physician can watch development of the follicle and determine if a woman is ovulating. Ultrasound is also used with injectable fertility drugs to make sure there are not too many eggs to avoid a pregnancy with higher-order multiples.

Hysterosalpingogram

A hysterosalpingogram (HSG) is a test that is done to determine if there is any blockage in the fallopian tubes. The test is done at a hospital or radiology lab. A thin catheter is inserted through the cervix and into the uterus. Dye is then sent up through the catheter to fill the tubes. The passage of the dye is observed through X-rays. If the dye can't get all the way through a tube, it could indicate blockage. The test can cause some cramping but is not very painful.

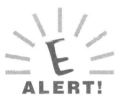
ALERT!

If you have polycystic ovarian syndrome (PCOS) and take the drug Metformin or Glucophage, be sure to tell your physician. The dye used in the HSG test can cause a reaction to this drug. Your physician will direct you to stop taking it for a few days.

There is some evidence that an HSG can clear mucous blockage from the tubes. A woman's fertility is increased in the months following an HSG.

Hysterosonography

Sometimes sterile saline will be injected into the uterine cavity, followed by pelvic ultrasound (hysterosonography). This enables the endocrinologist to check for uterine cavity shape, fibroids, or endometrial polyps. Hysterosonography may be used in addition to HSG.

Sperm Analysis

A sperm analysis is a normal part of any infertility workup. The male partner is asked to provide a sample of semen, in which the sperm is then counted and analyzed for mobility. Normally, the sample can be collected at home and brought into the lab. According to the American Society for Reproductive Medicine, male infertility contributes to 30 to 40 percent of infertile couples, so it is a factor that is always considered.

Endometrial Biopsy

If the physician suspects there is a problem with the development of the lining of the uterus (luteal phase defect, or LPD), a biopsy can be performed. A sample of endometrial tissue is taken in the doctor's office and is then analyzed. There are several different methods that can be used to take the sample.

Laparoscopy and Hysteroscopy

Laparoscopy is outpatient surgery performed with a small incision. A camera is inserted into the abdomen through the incision. This type of laparoscopy allows the physician to examine the uterus, ovaries, and tubes to determine if there is any abnormality.

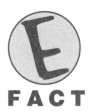

If you work with an endocrinologist, you may hear the term *ART*. This stands for *assisted reproductive technology* and refers to everything from fertility drugs to surrogacy.

A hysteroscopy is a camera passed through the cervix up into the uterus to examine the inside of the organ. These two procedures can be used as diagnostic tools but can also correct problems through surgery as well.

Fertility Drugs

There is no way to help a woman create more eggs than she has left, and there is no way to undo any aging that has happened to existing eggs. What doctors can do is help a woman ovulate regularly with the eggs she has left. Fertility drugs increase the number of eggs that mature each month, increasing the chances of pregnancy. A variety of drugs can be used, and your treatment will depend on your test results and your physician's evaluation of your situation. Clomid is the first line of attack. This is a pill you take at the beginning of your cycle to cause your ovaries to grow and release eggs. Other drugs are administered by injection and include gonadotropins, which stimulate egg production and their release.

Progesterone is a hormone that supports implantation of the egg in the uterus. Some women do not produce enough of this crucial hormone. It can be given in pill form to help promote implantation, but it is not technically a fertility drug.

Insemination

Insemination is generally the next step after a couple has tried fertility drugs. The physician monitors the woman's cycle. When she ovulates, her partner's sperm is collected and inserted directly into her uterus by way of a thin catheter. Placing the sperm directly into the uterus gives it a head start and increases the chances that the sperm will fertilize an egg and create a pregnancy.

If the woman's partner's sperm is determined not to be adequate, the couple can use a sperm donor and have the donated sperm inseminated.

In-Vitro Fertilization (IVF)

In-vitro fertilization is a process in which eggs are fertilized outside the uterus in a laboratory before being implanted. The woman undergoes hormone treatment to stimulate ovulation. Her eggs are then harvested using a needle. Her partner's sperm is collected and used to fertilize the eggs in the laboratory. Once the eggs are fertilized and observed, a few are selected and placed into the woman's uterus or tubes, depending on the days since fertilization. Additional embryos that are created can be frozen for later use.

Some women choose to use an egg donor if they do not have sufficient quantity or quality of eggs themselves. This is especially true in women over 40. Donors are young women, ideally in their 20s or early 30s. Donated eggs from young women have higher pregnancy rates and lower miscarriage rates.

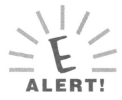

ALERT!

When you agree to undergo IVF treatment, you and your partner should carefully consider what you would like to have happen with unused embryos. They are usually frozen for later use, but if you never use them, you can destroy them, donate them for research, or donate them to other infertile couples. Deciding this up front can avoid confusion and waste later.

An egg donor takes fertility drugs to stimulate ovulation. Her eggs are then harvested and fertilized with your partner's sperm using IVF. The embryos can then be transferred to your uterus for the pregnancy. Any child you give birth to is legally yours, but it is still important to have documents drawn up by an attorney that waive the donor's rights. Egg donor programs may have long waiting lists. Using a known donor, such as a friend or relative, can bypass waiting but may raise parenting issues and have an impact on the families of both parties.

Surrogacy

Surrogacy is a process in which another woman carries a pregnancy for a woman or a woman and her partner. There are two types of surrogacy. In gestational surrogacy, the surrogate provides the egg, which is fertilized with the male partner's sperm. She then carries the pregnancy. In traditional surrogacy, the woman and her partner provide all the genetic material. Egg and sperm are united in a laboratory, and the embryos are then transferred to the surrogate who carries the pregnancy for them. The surrogate is not genetically related to the child in this method.

In any type of surrogacy arrangement, it is essential to have an experienced attorney represent you and handle the paperwork. State laws vary widely when it comes to surrogacy. In some states (Michigan, New Mexico, New York, and Washington) it is a crime to pay for surrogacy. In others, surrogacy contracts are unenforceable, though some states have laws permitting surrogacy contracts. California is the state that is friendliest to surrogacy.

The state has a specific court procedure set up to allow the prospective parents to have legal ties to their baby before it is born.

To find a surrogate, you can either work with an agency that specializes in surrogacy, or you can locate a potential surrogate on your own. It is very important that you have an attorney involved in each step of the process.

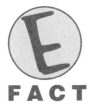

FACT

Surrogacy can cost from $25,000 to over $50,000, depending on the medical treatments necessary and the expenses permitted to be paid by the prospective parents in that state (some states permit the payment of living and other expenses for the surrogate).

New Options

Fertility begins to decline at a more rapid pace after the age of 37 or 38. Many women mistakenly think that they can defer childbearing until later in life and then successfully conceive with the help of artificial reproductive technology. In fact, age is the primary reason why infertility and pregnancy rates decline rapidly at this point even with artificial reproductive technology. Women who wish to defer pregnancy until after this age window or who wish to extend their fertility may have other options, though many of these are considered experimental at this time.

Two options are embryo cryopreservation and oocyte cryopreservation. Women who wish to defer pregnancy may, at a younger age, undergo ovarian stimulation, egg retrieval, and in-vitro fertilization with subsequent embryo freezing. Pregnancy success rates are 20 to 30 percent per transfer of two to three embryos. The drawback to this is that unless the woman already has a partner she wishes to conceive with at the time of in-vitro fertilization, the only other option is an anonymous sperm donor. Oocyte cryopreservation, in which a woman's ovaries are stimulated and her eggs are harvested and then frozen and preserved for future use, could theoretically overcome this obstacle, but pregnancy rates from this technology have been low to this point.

Staying Sane Through Fertility Treatments

Fertility treatments are a very emotional process, as well as a physical one. Not only are you coping with frustration and medical procedures, you may also be taking drugs that can affect your emotions. You're also coping with the fact that you are sharing a very private part of your life with physicians and nurses.

Stress has been shown to play an important part in infertility, so it's important to try to stay as calm and even-keeled as you can during treatments. Try to remind yourself about all the good things in your life. Focus on the things you enjoy and that give you pleasure. It is easy to get wrapped up in the ups and downs of each cycle. You absolutely must make time for yourself. While you will have to pay attention to important dates, you can't let your fertility treatments consume your entire life.

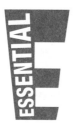

Everyone undergoing fertility treatments can use a little support. For information, a helpline, and support groups, contact RESOLVE: The National Infertility Association (*www.resolve.org*; 888-623-0744).

Remind yourself that other options are available if the treatments do not work, and just concentrate on living your life as it is. Enjoy what you have and love now instead of always focusing on what you don't have. There are many pathways to parenthood, and you will find your way.

Living a Child-free Life

Many men and women choose to live a life without children. Whether you come to this choice after considering other options or after facing obstacles on the pathway to parenthood, it is a viable choice. Many people live happy, fulfilled, and meaningful lives without becoming parents.

There are innumerable ways that do not include children to make a difference in the world, leave a legacy, share your love, and find meaning. If you come to this decision, you need to work to embrace and revel in the freedom it affords you instead of letting sorrow overtake you.

Chapter 4

Preconception Planning

Although getting pregnant is one of the most natural things in the world, you can do some things in advance to ensure that you will conceive quickly and have a healthy pregnancy. A little planning will help you reduce risks and feel prepared to become a mother.

Checkup

The American College of Obstetricians and Gynecologists (ACOG) now recommends that before you start trying to conceive, you see your gynecologist or gynecological nurse practitioner for a preconception checkup. This checkup not only allows her to do a thorough medical exam, it is also a good opportunity for you to talk to her about the best way to conceive quickly and to start a pregnancy in the best of health.

If possible, see your health-care provider six months before you begin trying to conceive. This will allow time to get any needed vaccinations, stop taking medications that could affect your pregnancy, and begin getting enough folic acid.

Medical History

An important part of the preconception exam is your medical history. Your health-care provider will want to get details on your medical and lifestyle history. He will also need information about your family health history, with a particular emphasis on any genetic diseases in your or your partner's family. Your health-care provider will be particularly interested in your menstrual history including length of periods, regularity, and when the last one occurred.

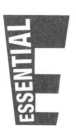

Before your preconception appointment, try to put together a complete family medical history, gathering information about how relatives died and any chronic or genetic diseases they had during their lives. It is easier to gather this information in advance than to try to rack your brain for it while sitting in the office.

Your health-care provider will want to know about any of the following in your history:

- Chronic diseases you have, such as asthma or diabetes
- Sexually transmitted diseases

- Pelvic inflammatory disease episodes
- Abnormal Pap smears
- Vaccination history
- Previous pregnancies, including ectopic, and ones that ended in miscarriage, stillbirth, and abortion
- Information about previous births, including type of delivery and any problems, including birth defects
- Previous surgeries you have had
- Your partner's health

Lifestyle

Your provider will probably ask you some questions about your lifestyle, including whether you drink or smoke or take any drugs (prescription, over the counter, or illegal). Your health-care provider may ask about a history of domestic violence or multiple partners. She may ask about what kind of exercise you get, and how often you get it, and your weight may be discussed if it is above or below average.

Your health-care provider may offer you some tips on figuring out your most fertile days each month and how often to have intercourse when you are trying to get pregnant. This is your opportunity to ask questions, so don't feel shy or embarrassed. Reproduction is an important part of life, and your health-care provider has lots of information that can be helpful to you.

Exam

The preconception checkup includes a urine sample and a recording of your height, weight, and blood pressure. Your health-care provider will do a pelvic exam, including a speculum examination of your cervix and vagina and a manual exam of your uterus, ovaries, and cervix. If you are due for a Pap smear, one will be taken. Your health-care provider may also take a similar smear to test for sexually transmitted diseases. A breast exam is also commonly part of the exam.

If you have not had or become immune to chicken pox and rubella (immunity can be checked with a blood test), you need to get vaccinated before conceiving since both of these diseases can have implications for your unborn child should you contract them. If you are at risk for hepatitis B, you should also be vaccinated for this.

Vitamins

A prenatal vitamin is recommended for women who are trying to conceive. The prenatal vitamin ensures that a woman's body can provide the appropriate nutrients to a growing fetus. Ideally, women should get a completely balanced diet from food, but unfortunately many women don't. A prenatal vitamin is good insurance even if you do eat well.

A prenatal vitamin is specially formulated to provide the vitamins and minerals in the correct amounts to support a pregnancy. If you've been taking a regular multivitamin, that's great, but you should switch to a prenatal vitamin while trying to conceive.

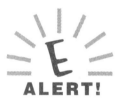

While you are trying to conceive, remember to tell your other physicians that you are trying to do so. For a certain time frame each month, you won't know if you are pregnant or not. During these days, you will want to avoid X-rays, certain drugs, and other treatments. Always request a pelvic shield for non-abdominal X-rays.

You can buy prenatal vitamins over the counter or you can get a prescription for them from your health-care provider. You might want to compare the prices of over-the-counter vitamins with your prescription co-pay to see which makes the most sense for you.

Folic Acid

One of the key components of a prenatal vitamin, and one of the most significant ways it differs from a simple multivitamin, is folic acid (also known as folate). The CDC recommends that women trying to conceive and those who are pregnant consume 400 micrograms (.4 mg) of folic acid daily. Although folic acid can also be obtained through fortified cereal and leafy green vegetables, the most reliable way to obtain this key nutrient is through a prenatal vitamin. Folic acid significantly reduces the risk of fetal neural tube defects that develop in the first few weeks of pregnancy. For this reason, all women who are trying to conceive need to ensure they get the right amount of folic acid, even before they think they might be pregnant.

Certain women may be at particular risk for having a baby with neural tube defects, particularly those who have a neural tube defect (or a partner with such a defect) or who have had a previous baby with a neural tube defect. However, there are many other circumstances where risk is increased. For those women, the dose of folic acid is higher at 4 mg per day. There is also evidence that preconception folic acid and prenatal vitamins may reduce the risk of having a baby with congenital heart disease.

Iron

Your prenatal vitamin will also make sure you get 30 mg of iron a day. Iron helps your body increase your blood supply during pregnancy. It is also essential because your baby needs to store iron to get him through his first few months of life.

Omega-3 DHA

Some health-care providers now recommend that women trying to conceive and those who are pregnant take omega-3 DHA fish oil supplements. This nutrient is important for fetal brain development. There are over-the-counter capsules specifically designed for pregnant women. These are free of mercury, a contaminant that sometimes appears in fish from polluted waters.

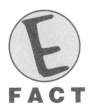

FACT

If you don't get enough iron in your diet or through vitamins, you can become anemic. Anemia can make you feel tired and look pale. Throughout your pregnancy, your doctor will check your blood to ensure you do not develop anemia. It is a good idea to build up your iron stores prior to pregnancy.

Calcium

Women over age 35 need to get 1000 mg of calcium per day during pregnancy. Dairy products, leafy green vegetables, and fortified orange juice are great sources. Prenatal vitamins also have calcium. If you are unable to obtain enough calcium in your diet (due to lactose intolerance, for instance), your doctor can prescribe a calcium supplement.

Drugs and Pre-Existing Conditions

At your preconception visit, you need to talk to your health-care provider about any chronic medical conditions you have and how they might affect your pregnancy. You also need to discuss any prescription medications you take, as well as over-the-counter drugs.

Medical Conditions

High blood pressure, diabetes, autoimmune diseases (such as rheumatoid arthritis or lupus), epilepsy, obesity, and asthma are all conditions that can be affected by pregnancy. They can also impact your pregnancy and the health of your baby. The good news is that most of the time, an experienced health-care provider can carefully manage any pre-existing conditions so that you can have a healthy and uneventful pregnancy.

Hypothyroidism (an underactive thyroid) is another important condition. Recent studies have shown that women with uncorrected hypothyroidism have an increased risk of having a baby with neurodevelopmental delay. This is even true of women who have subclinical hypothyroidism. In this case, blood tests show hypothyroidism even though the woman has no symptoms. This condition is fairly common in women, especially in older women. For this reason, the American Association of Clinical Endocrinologists recommends that women in the preconception period and in the first trimester of pregnancy be tested for hypothyroidism and that thyroid replacement medication be given when necessary. The American College of Obstetricians and Gynecologists (ACOG) has not endorsed this recommendation to date. However, in view of potential adverse effects on the baby, and the safety of thyroid replacement medication, it is probably a good idea to be tested, even if you don't have symptoms of hypothyroidism.

Drugs

If you are taking any prescription medications, you should bring a complete list to your preconception appointment. While some medications are not safe to take during pregnancy, others may be safe. You and your health-care provider may need to balance the risks and benefits before deciding what to do. In some cases you may be able to continue on your medication until you learn you are pregnant.

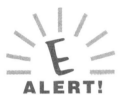

According the American Academy of Family Physicians, 10 percent of birth defects result from medications taken by the mother during pregnancy. Because of this, it is wise to avoid taking anything unless your doctor specifically approves it.

Talk to your health-care provider about over-the-counter medications. Most providers recommend that you avoid most of these while pregnant or trying to conceive, although acetaminophen (brand name Tylenol) and antacids are considered safe. In particular, you want to avoid ibuprofen (brand name Advil) and aspirin. Read the ingredients of over-the-counter medications carefully. Many contain alcohol and adrenaline-like substances. If you are not sure it is safe, ask your physician. The safety of most herbal remedies in pregnancy has not been studied and their safety is not certain. It is probably best to avoid these.

What to Avoid

It might seem strange that you need to start acting like you're pregnant when you first begin trying, but eliminating certain things from your diet and lifestyle before you're pregnant will give you the best chance for a healthy baby.

Caffeine

Caffeine is found in coffee, tea, chocolate, cocoa, cola, and some over-the-counter drugs. Large quantities of caffeine are linked to low birth-weight babies. Some studies show that small amounts of caffeine are safe, while others indicate that caffeine during pregnancy is not healthy for the baby. Each woman needs to make her own decision, in conjunction with her health-care provider, about whether to use caffeine and in what quantities. Some studies have shown that the miscarriage risk may be increased with high caffeine intake in women who have had several miscarriages in the past. These women may wish to avoid caffeine. It is important to know that drip coffee has the highest caffeine level, with perked and instant having less. As with all things, moderation is probably the key.

Alcohol

No amount of alcohol has been proven to be safe during pregnancy. Alcohol enters your bloodstream and travels through the umbilical cord to the baby. Alcohol is known to slow the baby's growth, cause birth defects, and alter brain development.

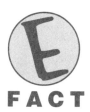

FACT

Fetal alcohol spectrum disorders (previously called fetal alcohol syndrome) can occur in children whose mothers drink alcohol during pregnancy. The result for the baby is disfiguration of facial features and central nervous system disorders. Because of the dangers of these disorders, women are advised to avoid all alcohol during pregnancy and while trying to conceive.

Fish

While fish is considered an essential part of a healthy diet, many fish have dangerous levels of mercury, making them unsafe to eat while pregnant or trying to conceive. The fish to avoid are the following:

- Shark
- Swordfish
- King mackerel
- Tilefish (also called golden or white snapper)

White or albacore tuna and tuna steak also have high levels of mercury and because of this, more than six ounces per week is not considered safe. In general, pregnant women or women trying to conceive should limit themselves to no more than two servings of fish (twelve ounces total) per week. Shrimp, salmon, pollock, catfish, and light tuna contain the lowest levels of mercury. If you want to consume fish from local waters, consult your state environmental department for advice on what is safe.

Soft Cheeses

The CDC recommends that pregnant women and women who are attempting to conceive should avoid unpasteurized soft cheeses, including Brie, Camembert, queso fresco, queso blanco, feta, and goat cheese. When they are made from unpasteurized milk, soft cheeses can contain listeria, a bacteria which can be dangerous to the developing baby. Listeria is also found in unpasteurized farm milk. Check the label before buying cheeses.

Deli and Uncooked Meats

Deli meats are another possible source for listeria and because of this, it is recommended that pregnant women not consume ready-to-eat deli meats unless they are heated to 160 degrees (or steaming). Refrigerated patés and meat spreads should be avoided, as should refrigerated seafood spreads and smoked seafood, unless they are heated through. Raw or rare meat can carry the toxoplasmosis parasite, which can cause birth defects.

Chemicals

If you work near or around hazardous chemicals such as solvents, it is important to discuss this with your doctor and get details about the chemicals from your employer. Certain chemicals can increase the risk of miscarriage or birth defects and must be avoided by pregnant women or those trying to conceive. It may be possible to continue working if ventilation is good and facemasks are used.

Other Dangers

There are other things to be aware of and be careful about while you are trying to get pregnant and while you are pregnant. Here are a few:

- **Cat litter:** If you have a cat, someone else should change the litter box because of the danger of toxoplasmosis. Petting your cat or having other contact is not dangerous.
- **Child care:** If you work in a day care center, wash your hands or wear gloves when changing diapers or handling toys that are mouthed. Cytomegalovirus (CMV) is shared through urine and saliva and can have serious effects on the unborn baby.
- **Hot tubs and spas:** The elevated temperatures can impair fertility and create problems for the baby if you are pregnant.

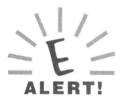
ALERT!

Pregnant women may be at higher risk for serious complications from influenza. The CDC recommends that all women who will, are, or may be pregnant during flu season (generally mid-November to end of March) receive the flu shot. It can be given anytime during pregnancy.

Starting at a Healthy Weight

Your health-care provider will discuss your weight at your preconception checkup. If you are over- or underweight, she will probably advise you to try to get your weight within a healthy range before trying to get pregnant.

Being underweight or overweight can make it more difficult to get pregnant and can also affect your chances for a healthy pregnancy. To find out a healthy weight for your body, you need to figure out your body mass index (BMI). Divide your weight in pounds by your height in inches squared. Take this subtotal and multiply it by 703. This is your BMI. Next, you need to determine where your BMI falls within these ranges:

- 18.5 or less: Underweight
- 18.5 to 24.9: Normal
- 25.0 to 29.9: Overweight
- 30.0 to 39.9: Obese
- 40 or greater: Extremely obese

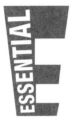

You can use the online calculator or chart at *www.consumer.gov/weight loss/bmi.htm* to determine your BMI. Your doctor will most likely have a chart in the office for your reference.

Some women feel frustrated when their physician recommends waiting to become pregnant until they are at a healthy weight. If you are close to your ideal weight, taking a month or two to reach it may not be a problem. But if you are worried that time is running out on your fertility, talk to your doctor about how your weight can be managed during pregnancy so that you can get started trying immediately.

Exercise

Continuing your regular exercise program while you try to conceive should not pose a problem, but it is a good idea to discuss it with your physician. Exercise is an important component to a healthy pregnancy, and when done before and during pregnancy it reduces the risk of preterm labor.

Genetic Counseling

Genetic counseling is a process in which you and your partner's risks for passing on genetic diseases are evaluated. A genetic counselor is a specially trained health-care professional who is trained to interpret and evaluate genetic risks.

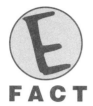

Approximately 3 percent of all babies born in the United States have a birth defect. There are 4,000 known types of birth defects, which lead to physical abnormalities and problems. Many types, however, can be cured or treated.

Genetic counseling is recommended for all women over age 35 and especially for women who have these additional risk factors:

- An abnormal prenatal test result
- A defect identified through an amniocentesis result
- A close family member with an inherited genetic disease
- A child with a genetic disease or birth defect (or a partner who has such a child)
- Ethnicity associated with high rates of certain genetic diseases (such as African Americans and sickle cell anemia)

When you meet with a genetic counselor, she will take a detailed family history. The counselor may arrange or coordinate testing such as blood work or amniocentesis. She then will help you understand how your family history could impact your child and what the risks are of various disorders, diseases, and defects. She will discuss how to interpret test results and how to make a decision based on those test results. When you have test results, if there is one that is of concern, your genetic counselor will coordinate with your physician and help you understand the results.

Understanding Your Cycle

Understanding how your cycle works will help you learn your most fertile times each month and allow you to capitalize on those times. Getting pregnant takes some organizational skill. The average woman has a menstrual cycle that lasts twenty-eight to thirty-two days. If your cycle is longer or shorter, it doesn't mean you can't get pregnant, but it does mean you need to have a good understanding of your cycle.

Cycle Basics

The menstrual cycle has several distinct phases. The first phase is the follicular phase, when an egg is growing to maturity. This starts on the first day of your period and lasts five to seven days. Around day fourteen of the cycle (or fourteen days before the start of your next period), ovulation occurs. An egg is released and begins to travel down the fallopian tubes. This part of your cycle is called the luteal phase. If on this journey a sperm fertilizes the egg, it will travel to the uterus and seek to implant in the wall of the uterus. If the egg is not fertilized, it will disintegrate and be discharged when the lining of the uterus begins to shed, beginning another period. If your cycle is longer or shorter than average, your ovulation probably won't be on day fourteen, but instead will be about fourteen days before your next period is due.

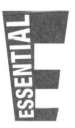

Women over age 35 take on average between one and two years to get pregnant. That may seem like a long time, but if you carefully track your cycles, maximize your fertile times, and stay positive, you can improve your odds.

Your most fertile period is one to two days before you ovulate (giving the sperm time to make the journey and wait for the egg), during ovulation, and one day afterward. This is actually a fairly small window and can be hard to pinpoint if you don't know when you are ovulating. Because of this, you will probably want to try to track when exactly you are ovulating. There are several methods you can use to do this.

Basal Body Temperature

Your basal body temperature is your temperature taken first thing in the morning, at about the same time every day, before you get up and move around. When you are ovulating, it will rise slightly. To monitor this temperature, buy a digital thermometer and download a graph from *http://www.4woman.gov/pregnancy/tools/bbt-chart-blank.pdf* or make your own using graph paper. Take your temperature each morning and record it. Your preovulation temperature will be around 96 to 98 degrees Fahrenheit. When you ovulate, it should rise .4 to .8 degrees and remain heightened until you get your period. If you are pregnant, it should continue to stay higher.

Your basal body temperature is affected and may appear to rise if you do or experience any of the following:

- Have a fever
- Drink alcohol the night before
- Smoke cigarettes the night before
- Toss and turn or don't sleep well
- Get up to go to the bathroom before you take it
- Have a conversation before you take it
- Have intercourse before you take it

The problem with basal body temperature charting is that your temperature does not rise until after you ovulate, and your most fertile period is right before, during, and right after ovulation. However, if you chart it every month, you will begin to get a sense for what day of the month you will most likely ovulate and will be able to predict in advance when it will occur.

To do basal body charting successfully, keep the thermometer, pencil, and chart on your nightstand. Make it a habit that the first thing you do each morning when you open your eyes is to take your temperature. It takes less than a minute, depending on the speed of your thermometer, and can quickly become part of your morning routine.

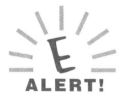

While you may think that more sex will increase your odds of conceiving, it is actually better to have intercourse about every other day during your fertile period, to allow your partner's sperm reserve to build back up.

Keep these charts, even for months in which you do not conceive, because they can help your doctor understand your cycle and possible problems. If you do conceive, the chart will help pinpoint when exactly it happened.

Cervical Mucous

As eggs mature, they cause more estrogen to be released in the woman's body. Estrogen causes the lining of the uterus to thicken (so that a fertilized egg can implant) and also causes the mucous produced by the cervix to change and become friendlier to sperm. By monitoring the changes in the cervical mucous, you can determine where in your cycle you are. Once an egg is about to be or has just been released, cervical mucous becomes clear, slippery, and stretchy, like raw egg whites, and also increases in amount. On nonfertile days, mucous may be white and cloudy, or clear but sticky.

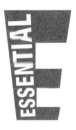

Home ovulation test kits predict your ovulation one to two days in advance, giving you some advance notice. These tests are considered very accurate and are simple to do. When they are used in conjunction with basal body temperature charts and cervical mucous tests, they can greatly improve your odds of getting pregnant because you will have the most information possible.

To check your cervical mucous, you can insert a finger into your vagina, remove it, then touch that finger with another to see if the mucous stretches between them. You can also examine the discharged mucous on a piece of toilet paper. You may want to note these changes on your basal body temperature chart so that you can have all your information in one place.

Your Partner's Health

Because your partner is providing half of the material needed to create your baby, his health is important as well. Doctors don't do preconception check-ups for men, but there are steps your partner can take to help improve your odds of conceiving and having a healthy pregnancy.

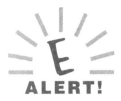

ALERT!

Some prescription drugs can adversely affect sperm development, so if your partner is taking any prescriptions, he should check with his physician about possible side effects before you start trying to conceive.

Men who wish to become fathers should stop smoking and drinking alcohol. They should also reduce or eliminate their exposure to hazardous chemicals in the workplace. To maximize your chances of conception, your partner may want to take steps to maintain a proper temperature in his testes, such as not wearing tight underwear and limiting the use of a laptop computer directly on his lap. Increased heat can lead to sperm defects, so maintaining a proper temperature is key.

You should also talk to your partner about his use of hot baths, hot tubs, or saunas. High temperatures can inhibit the ability of sperm to function. Fortunately men make sperm constantly, but constant exposure of the testicles to high temperatures may reduce fertility.

Chapter 5

Staying Healthy During Pregnancy

Pregnancy is a wonderful time, but it is also busy. You're preparing to add a new person to your family; first, you must get the new person fully grown and ready to be born. Taking care of yourself during pregnancy should be your number-one priority.

Weight Gain and Nutrition

Weight gain during pregnancy may be something you dread or look forward to. Either way, it is an important part of ensuring that your baby will be healthy. More than packing on pounds, weight gain is about proper nutrition and a healthy diet.

How Much Weight to Gain

Current weight-gain recommendations for an average woman are between twenty-five and thirty-five pounds over the course of a pregnancy. Women who are underweight will need to gain more, and women who are overweight will need to gain less. The key is that you do need to gain weight. Each woman should consult with her own health-care provider about how much weight is right for her to gain in pregnancy.

In general, weight gain should be spread out so that you gain three to five pounds total in the first trimester, then one to two pounds per week after that. Weight gain should be slow and steady. Pregnancy is not the time to begin a diet, but it is the time to have a healthy diet.

Where the Weight Goes

Weight gain during pregnancy fortunately does not go straight to your hips. Instead, it is used in a variety of ways to help your baby grow and assist your body in changing. The weight gain is distributed as follows:

- **12 pounds:** Placenta
- **7 to 8 pounds:** Baby
- **7 pounds:** Fats and nutrients
- **4 pounds:** Increased blood volume
- **4 pounds:** Fluid retention
- **2 pounds:** Amniotic fluid
- **2 pounds:** Uterus
- **2 pounds:** Breast tissue

A Healthy Diet

Pregnant women require an additional 300 calories per day during pregnancy, and possibly more depending on how much they are exercising. 300 calories isn't much, and the concept of "eating for two" doesn't really hold true. It is usually recommended that pregnant women eat three small meals and two or three snacks throughout the day. Eating more frequently can help relieve nausea and keep you from getting overly hungry.

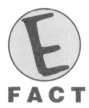

FACT

Many women spend a lot of time stressing out about pregnancy weight gain. If they aren't gaining quite enough, they are terrified of starving their baby. If they gain a little too much, they are certain they will be fat forever. Aim for the amount your doctor recommends, but if you're a couple pounds off in either direction, don't make yourself crazy.

A healthy diet includes the following:

- 2 to 4 servings of fruit
- 3 to 5 servings of vegetables
- 6 to 11 servings of grains
- 3 to 4 servings of protein
- 3 to 4 servings of dairy products

The thing to remember during pregnancy is to make every calorie count, as much as you are able. Potato chips provide very few nutrients for your baby, but a fruit smoothie, apple slices, or raisins help your baby grow. Pregnancy is a time for conscious eating. While it's okay to indulge yourself once in a while, your goal should be to eat food that has value.

Eating three small meals and two or three snacks, as most experts recommend, might mean adjusting your routine. This is particularly true if you are working or are used to having a large evening meal with your partner. Listen to your body. If you're hungry, eat. If eating does not appeal to you, don't eat at that time.

Exercise

Gone are the days when pregnant women were expected to just put their feet up. Staying active and getting exercise is a key part of a healthy pregnancy. Always check with your health-care provider before doing any exercise during pregnancy to make sure the type and amount you're doing is safe for you.

The Importance of Exercise

Exercise is important during pregnancy because it helps keep both mother and baby healthy. Exercise during pregnancy also helps keep your body functioning well and can prevent common pregnancy problems such as constipation, varicose veins, back pain, and general fatigue. One study showed that exercising before or during pregnancy reduced the risk of developing preeclampsia (a dangerous high-blood-pressure condition), with the risk decreasing the more frequent and intense the exercise was. Exercise also has mental health benefits and can keep you feeling positive about your body and in control of your pregnancy.

Studies looking at exercise during pregnancy have shown that it has no negative effects on the baby's birth weight or on a higher incidence of small-for-gestational age or growth-restricted babies. In fact, one study showed that weight-bearing exercise begun in the first trimester of pregnancy actually increased neonatal birth weight and lean body mass—in other words, the babies were not just "fat"—as well as enhancing placental growth.

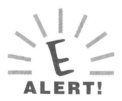

ALERT!

It is important to stay hydrated during exercise while pregnant because you can lose one or two quarts of water per hour when exercising. Drink water during and after exercise. Wear cool, comfortable clothing that moves easily and does not constrain your pregnant belly.

Exercise will also help your body prepare for labor and delivery. There are prenatal exercise classes specifically designed for pregnant women given through local hospitals or fitness centers. You can also purchase DVDs and books about exercise during pregnancy. Staying active and fit will keep your endurance and strength up and help prepare your body for birth.

Recommendations

The American College of Obstetricians and Gynecologists (ACOG) recommends that most pregnant women get thirty minutes of moderate exercise on most days. This can be achieved in one large block of time, for example, thirty minutes of swimming, or in smaller blocks of time, such as taking three ten-minute walks at different points during the day. Almost all types of exercise are safe during pregnancy, except contact sports and impact exercise.

If you did not exercise regularly before pregnancy and you want to start now, it is important to start slowly and gradually. You can't suddenly do thirty minutes a day of walking or tennis if you didn't do so before you were pregnant. You might want to start with ten minutes of exercise every other day, build up to once a day, then increase the time from there.

ACOG recommends the following when it comes to exercise:

- Skip contact sports or those that could cause mild impact to your pregnant belly, such as soccer.
- Avoid exercise where there is a risk of falling, such as horseback riding.
- Never attempt to scuba dive while pregnant because of the risk of decompression.
- After the first trimester, do not do any exercises that require you to be on your back.
- Stay away from exercises that require jerky or bouncy movements, which can put a strain on your muscles.
- Avoid exercising at high altitudes.

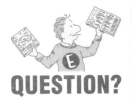

Why is 35 the age at which you suddenly are an "older mother"?
It might seem like an arbitrary number (why not 34 or 36?) but 35 is the age at which the risk of performing an amniocentesis is the same as the chances of having a baby with Down syndrome, so that is the age at which it became sensible to consider amniocentesis for all women.

Nausea

Nausea or morning sickness bothers many women during pregnancy, with up to 80 percent experiencing nausea and 50 percent vomiting. Although it's called morning sickness, it can happen at any time of the day. There is some good news, however. One large study from the Swedish National Birth Registry showed that older women were less likely to report morning sickness in the first trimester than their younger counterparts.

Morning sickness is thought to be caused by the many changes your body is going through, particularly the hormonal changes. It's most common in the first trimester, and most women can expect the symptoms to end by the time they are in their second trimester. Unfortunately some women experience nausea throughout their pregnancies. But fewer women who have morning sickness have miscarriages, so being sick does have its benefits.

Nausea is not fun, but it's not dangerous unless you become dehydrated or lose weight. Becoming dehydrated actually makes morning sickness worse, so it is important to stay hydrated even when the last thing you feel like doing is drinking. Eating small, frequent meals can also help hold off nausea, since some women find that hunger can be a trigger.

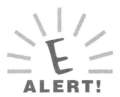

Call your health-care provider if you are unable to keep fluids down, are dizzy, vomiting frequently, have a decrease in urination or very dark urine, feel dehydrated, have headaches, feel confused, or have rapid heartbeats. These are signs of hyperemesis, a severe form of morning sickness that requires immediate treatment.

There are some other things that can help lessen morning sickness. Ginger has been shown to help, so ginger tea or lollipops may be a solution. Getting enough sleep, avoiding strong odors, skipping food that is greasy or spicy, eating and drinking at different times, eating cold food, eating something salty at the beginning of a meal, and eating enough protein can all help quell nausea.

Sleep Difficulties

Although pregnancy is a time when your body is working hard, it may be a time when you have difficulty sleeping well. Making sure you get enough rest can help you feel better throughout your pregnancy.

Sleeping difficulties are common throughout pregnancy for different reasons. In early pregnancy, nausea can make sleep difficult, but many women also find they are very fatigued even if they sleep a normal amount at night. Make time to rest when your body needs to. Insomnia is very common during pregnancy. It tends to be worse in the first and third trimesters. In the first trimester, pregnancy hormones such as progesterone cause sleepiness and fatigue. This often prompts the pregnant woman to take frequent naps during the day and makes it hard to fall asleep at night. The lesson to be learned here is to rest throughout the day without napping a lot.

Sleep gets increasingly uncomfortable as pregnancy progresses because of the size of your belly, but also because of the need to frequently urinate. In the third trimester, the baby and growing uterus are usually responsible for the discomfort that causes insomnia. Sleeping with a lot of pillows, such as body pillows, can make late pregnancy nights more restful.

Exercise and caffeine avoidance may also help insomnia. In most cases, pregnancy insomnia can be managed without medications. Occasionally medications such as Benadryl can be used, but it is probably best to try and do without sleep medications.

In women who are morbidly obese, insomnia or sleep disturbance may be a sign of sleep apnea, a potentially serious disorder in which the sleeper stops breathing for several seconds. Sleep apnea is harmful over time and actually may be detrimental to the baby during pregnancy. Sleep studies are generally required to diagnose the condition, and special oxygen treatment during sleep is required.

Your mind may also interfere with your sleep. You may be worrying about your job, how you will manage a baby and a career, as well having concerns about your baby's risk for problems. Try to look at your concerns rationally, and do everything you can to solve them during the day. Make nighttime a worry-free time. Do things that will relax you before bedtime, such as reading, taking a bath, or asking your partner for a massage.

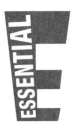

Sleeping in whatever position you are comfortable in is fine until about twenty-four weeks. After this point, sleeping on your back is not recommended since the weight of your uterus can compress arteries and reduce blood flow to the baby.

Aches and Pains

Because your body changes so much during pregnancy, you're likely to experience some discomfort at some point along the way. Remember that these pains are temporary and just another reminder that you have a little person who will soon join your life.

Fatigue

Pregnancy makes you tired. Period. Your body is working hard to grow and support a new life, and that takes a lot of energy. Older mothers may find that they are more fatigued than they expected, and pregnancy does tend to get more tiring the older you are.

You have to listen to what your body is telling you each day of your pregnancy. If you are tired, you need to find a way to rest. This can be difficult, especially if you're trying to stay on top of things at work now to make things easier when you take time off for the birth. Even a ten-minute cat nap at your desk can help you get through the day. Look for ways to make things easier for yourself. Sit whenever possible. Ask your partner to handle the errands or chores you normally do. Take every opportunity you can to ease the burden on yourself.

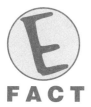

Getting enough sleep may help shorten your labor and avoid a cesarean section. A study from the University of California at San Francisco showed that women who got less than six hours of sleep in late pregnancy had longer labors and were 4.5 times more likely to have a C-section. Women who got six to seven hours of shuteye were 3.7 times more likely to have a C-section.

Eating well will also help with fatigue. Eating small snacks throughout the day will help keep your energy levels high. Thinking positively and working to avoid fatigue rather than cope with it once it arrives can also help.

Pain and Discomfort

It's pretty outrageous to think that nature has arranged for women to carry a six- or seven-pound baby around inside of them. Sometimes during pregnancy you feel like an overstuffed suitcase. Every pregnant woman experiences some discomfort, but you don't have to be miserable the entire nine months.

Back pain is common in late pregnancy. There are some things you can do to lessen any discomfort you're experiencing. If wearing high heels makes your back hurt, stop wearing them. Comfortable shoes will make your back, feet, and legs feel much happier. Sit in comfortable chairs that give good back support. Avoid sitting or standing in one position for too long. Learn to do some simple exercises to help strengthen your back. (You can ask your health-care provider, try out a pregnancy exercise class or DVD, or, if your pain is severe, see a physical therapist.) Avoid heavy lifting.

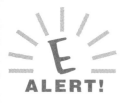

During pregnancy, your body produces a hormone called relaxin, which helps relax your pelvic joints so that giving birth will be easier. Unfortunately, this hormone also causes joints in other areas of your body to loosen, causing back pain, groin pain, and other discomfort during pregnancy.

Swelling in the hands, legs, and feet is another common pregnancy problem that is called edema. Mild swelling is normal, especially in the ankles, and is nothing to be concerned about. Swelling occurs when your body retains more water, and the excess fluid collects in your extremities. Call your health-care provider if you notice very sudden or extreme swelling or swelling elsewhere, such as your face, or if you experience rapid weight gain (five pounds per week or more). This could be a sign of preeclampsia. Taking water pills or diuretics will not reduce swelling in pregnancy and is potentially harmful.

Elevate your swollen legs or feet to help make them feel better. Crossing your legs will make the swelling worse, as will tight socks or knee-high or thigh-high stockings. If your hands swell, elevate them on pillows next to you. Frequent movements and stretching can also help reduce swelling as can drinking a lot of water. There is no need to restrict your salt intake during pregnancy through a low-sodium diet; however, excessive intake of salt and salty foods will definitely make the swelling worse.

Nasal congestion is another common pregnancy complaint. As your blood volume increases, it causes your nasal passages to swell. A cool-mist humidifier can help you breathe easier. If part of your congestion is allergy related, your physician may prescribe nasal sprays, some of which contain steroids. These are safe during pregnancy under medical supervision. However, some over-the-counter nasal sprays contain adrenaline-like drugs; these should be avoided as they can have effects on the blood flow to the uterus. You may also experience bloody noses more frequently during pregnancy and bleeding from the gums when you brush your teeth. However, if either of these become excessive or are accompanied by bruising or blood in places such as the urine, you should consult your physician.

Constipation

The pregnancy hormone progesterone slows down your digestive tract and thus is to blame for the constipation that many pregnant women experience. Late in pregnancy, the weight of the uterus can also press on the rectum, causing constipation. Constipation is something you can manage by drinking lots of water, exercising, and eating high fiber foods. If you can't seem to get it under control, talk to your health-care provider about the amount of iron in your prenatal vitamin; too much iron can cause constipation. You may also be able to take an over-the-counter fiber supplement or stool softeners. Laxatives, however, should not be taken.

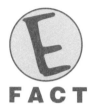

FACT

While pregnancies over age 35 do carry some additional risks, they may actually be healthier than a younger woman's. If a 35-year-old woman eats well, exercises, does not smoke or drink, and gains the recommended amount of weight, she has a much greater chance of having a healthy pregnancy than a 24-year-old who drinks, smokes, gains too little or too much weight, and does not exercise.

If constipation leads to straining to have a bowel movement it can cause or worsen hemorrhoids, which are enlarged varicose veins in the rectal area. Alternating hot and warm packs or water in a bath can help. Ask your health-care provider to recommend an over-the-counter treatment if needed. Rectal bleeding from hemorrhoids is a common complaint. Generally, rectal bleeding of this kind follows a bowel movement, is bright red, and is found on toilet paper after wiping. If the rectal bleeding does not follow this pattern, if you are not sure the blood is coming from the rectum (instead of the vagina), or if you are concerned, you should call your health-care provider.

Heartburn

The hormone progesterone, again, is responsible for heartburn. This hormone causes the valve between your esophagus and stomach to relax during pregnancy. Stomach acid can bubble up into the esophagus, creating that burning feeling in your throat and chest. For the same reason, women who have pre-existing gastroesophageal reflux (GERD) may experience a worsening of their symptoms during pregnancy. During the third trimester, the enlarging uterus also adds pressure, pushing the stomach upward. Eating smaller meals can help relieve heartburn. You should also avoid greasy and fatty foods. In addition, nicotine, caffeine, and peppermint further relax the esophageal sphincter, worsening the symptoms. Avoid lying down within an hour of eating and try to limit greasy and spicy foods that can aggravate heartburn. If these steps do not alleviate the symptoms, antacids may be helpful. Ask your health-care provider before taking any over-the-counter antacids. Generally, they can be taken thirty minutes after meals and at bedtime.

Emotional Ups and Downs

Many women expect pregnancy to be a time of sheer joy. In reality, it is often a time of ups and downs. This is due in part to the physical changes you are going through and in part to the major changes in your entire life.

Stay Focused

Staying focused on the end result of your pregnancy will help you weather the emotions and physical discomforts. Remind yourself that before you know it, your baby will have arrived. It's perfectly okay not to adore being pregnant. While there are women who love it, there are just as many who don't enjoy it at all. The good thing about pregnancy is that above all else, it is only temporary.

Give Up Control

During pregnancy, your body may seem to have a mind of its own. You aren't and will never be the same, so expecting yourself to feel and act the same as always is not realistic. Instead, let pregnancy take you on its journey, and try to enjoy what it gives you. You will probably experience very intense emotions that are different from anything you've felt before. This isn't necessarily a bad thing and instead opens you up to the intensity of motherhood.

There are simply going to be days when you feel tired, scared, joyful, frustrated, or cranky during pregnancy. And sometimes there will be nothing you can do to change that, so the easiest thing is to give yourself a break and just ride it through.

Chapter 6

How an Over-35 Pregnancy Is Managed

You may be a bit nervous or concerned about finding a health-care provider you're comfortable with and getting details about how exactly your pregnancy will be monitored and cared for and whether there are differences because of your age. The good news is that most OB/GYNs, nurse-midwives, and maternal-fetal medicine specialists are very well versed in caring for older mothers. Your role as a patient though is to be involved, ask questions, and follow the good advice you receive.

Deciding on a Health-Care Provider

Because there are a variety of different approaches and patient needs, there are a variety of health-care providers you can choose to care for you during your pregnancy and delivery. Keep in mind that you are able to switch to a different provider during your pregnancy if your needs change.

Family Physician

A family physician is trained to handle pregnancy and delivery. If you have a family physician you see for the rest of your health care and feel comfortable with, you may want to continue to see her for pregnancy care. You should ask if she has had additional training in obstetrics beyond her family physician training. The advantage with family physicians is that they can treat pregnancy as part of the larger picture of your overall health and may also be able to treat your child once he is born.

Most family physicians are not able to do C-sections (according to the American Academy of Family Physicians, only 4.1 percent of its members do so). Many family physicians will refer a woman over age 35 to an obstetrician or maternal-fetal medicine specialist, but this varies with the family physician's training level. Family physicians attend 20 percent of U.S. births. In general, if everything about your pregnancy is low risk, your family physician may continue to care for you.

Most family physicians have at least one or two OB/GYNs with whom they regularly work and consult. Family physicians must have obstetrical backup as part of their hospital privilege requirements. It is probably wise to ask your family doctor about her obstetrical backup and whom she may consult if you develop problems during labor or develop a pregnancy problem.

Obstetrician

Most obstetricians are actually OB/GYNs, meaning they care for women's reproductive systems in general (gynecology) as well as handling pregnancies (obstetrics). If you already see your OB/GYN for yearly visits, you may decide you are comfortable continuing to see her for your pregnancy care. Many obstetricians consult with a maternal-fetal medicine specialist about patients who are over 35, sending the patient to the specialist for ultrasound and other diagnostic tests. Patients who are at high risk may be transferred completely to a maternal-fetal medicine specialist.

Maternal-Fetal Medicine Specialist

Also called a perinatologist, a maternal-fetal medicine specialist is an obstetrician who has completed an additional two to three years of fellowships after the obstetrical residency that follows medical school. Maternal-fetal medicine specialists provide care for the mother and developing baby in pregnancies that are considered complicated. This kind of specialist may take over the care of the pregnancy or consult with an obstetrician, midwife, or family physician about the pregnancy, including performing ultrasounds and other diagnostic tests.

Midwife

There are several types of midwives. A certified nurse-midwife is a nurse who has been trained and licensed to deliver babies. A certified midwife has completed training and licensing but does not have a nursing degree. There are also midwives who are not certified or licensed. Different states have different requirements and standards for unlicensed midwives.

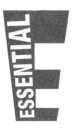

For more information about midwives, or to locate one in your area, contact the American College of Nurse-Midwives (*www.acnm.org*), a professional organization; or Citizens for Midwifery (*www.cfmidwifery. org*), a grassroots organization dedicated to providing information.

Midwives often work as part of a larger obstetrical practice. All midwives should have an obstetrician they can consult with and to whom they can refer patients. Midwives have at least one or two OB/GYNs with whom they regularly work and consult. Midwives who deliver in hospitals must have obstetrical backup as part of their hospital privilege requirements. It is probably wise to ask your midwife about her obstetrical backup and who she may consult if you develop problems during labor or develop a pregnancy problem.

Midwives cannot perform C-sections. Midwives deliver babies in hospitals, birth centers, and at home births. Some women prefer midwives because they feel they get more personal attention and a more natural approach. Should a complication occur during a midwife-assisted birth, you will be transferred to a hospital (if you are not already in one) and cared for by a physician.

Home births are a controversial area in obstetrics, and most states have laws governing home deliveries. The pregnancy should be low risk; many would argue that advanced maternal age alone is a risk factor that would preclude home birth. You should make sure that the midwife handling a home birth is in compliance with state regulations, is complying with safe guidelines to determine pregnancy risk, is licensed in the state he or she practices in, and has an obstetrical backup and plan should problems arise.

Doula

A doula is a birth assistant who provides support, encouragement, comfort measures, and companionship to a mother during labor. Doulas are trained in assisting women and their families through the birth process. Some statistics show that a woman supported by a doula is likely to have a shorter labor and is less likely to have a C-section, epidural, forceps delivery, or augmented labor. A doula is not able to deliver the baby or provide prenatal care. You can use a doula in addition to your physician or midwife if you choose. To find a doula, you can contact Doulas of North America (DONA) at *www.dona.org*.

Finding a Health-Care Provider

Once you've decided what kind of health-care provider you want to work with during your pregnancy and for your birth, you need to actually find one with whom you feel comfortable. Get a few names and then meet with several providers to determine which one is right for you.

To obtain names to consider, talk to friends and family or ask your primary-care provider or gynecologist. You can also get a list of participating providers from your health-insurance company. Another option is to contact an organization such as the American College of Obstetricians and Gynecologists (*www.acog.org*) or the American College of Nurse-Midwives (*www.acnm.org*) for referrals to providers in your area.

Once you have some names, you may wish to check with your state medical board to determine if there are any grievances against the provider. Next, make an appointment with your top three picks. Go to the appointment with a list of questions that will help you determine how well the provider meets your needs. You may want to ask about things like these:

- Hospitals or birth centers where the provider delivers
- Costs
- Insurance accepted
- Other providers in the practice and on-call coverage
- C-section rates
- Episiotomy rates
- Whether there is a different approach taken for women over 35
- Availability of prenatal appointment times and dates

If the provider is a midwife, you should also find out what doctors are associated with the practice and how available they are should they be needed.

Another important factor when choosing an obstetrical caretaker, specifically a physician, is credentials. Many states have Web sites that document a physician's credentials, education, board certification, and years in training. Litigation history is also generally available. Just because a physician has been sued does not imply incompetence. In some cases a physician's malpractice insurance company may decide to settle a lawsuit for financial reasons only, since the settlement may well be less than the cost of defending the case. However, multiple suits in a short period of time with large settlements may suggest a problem. In addition, temporary loss of license, restriction of practice, or probation may be warning signs.

Board certification is an important topic. Midwifery, obstetrics and gynecology, family medicine, and maternal-fetal medicine all have certification processes. Young physicians who are only a few years out of residency training may not yet have their certification since it takes several years to achieve. They may be excellent physicians; you should inquire if they are in a group practice or have a more experienced colleague available should they run into difficulty.

In obstetrics and maternal-fetal medicine, most physicians achieve board certification within three to five years after residency or fellowship training, respectively. Most medical boards now issue time-limited certifications, requiring some form of recertification every six to ten years. Board certification is not a guarantee of good care. However, if a physician who has been out of training for some time does not have her board certification, it may raise some red flags.

Planning Your Medical Care

Medical care, like any other important part of your life, is something you should plan. You should have an understanding of how your pregnancy will be managed and cared for and what your role in the process is.

There are a variety of things you will want to know about your pregnancy care, such as the following:

- How often you will have prenatal appointments
- What you need to bring to each appointment
- What types of testing you will need and when in your pregnancy it will be scheduled
- What kinds of payments you will be responsible for and when they will be due
- Who you will see at your appointments, and if you will get to see all the providers in the practice
- What steps you personally need to take to ensure you have a healthy pregnancy
- What warning signs to watch for, both at your current stage of pregnancy and in the future

Once you have the answers to these questions, you will be able to form a complete timetable in your mind of what will happen and when throughout your pregnancy. You will feel calmer and more in control because you understand what your health-care provider is planning and what you need to do every step of the way.

Asking Questions and Educating Yourself

Your health-care provider is a medical expert and is trained to suggest options for your care. Still, you make the decisions and are in control of your own body. Because of this, it is very important that you work with your health-care provider, ask questions, and educate yourself.

While your health-care provider tries to offer the information you need, often questions and concerns come up that have not been addressed. At every appointment, make a point to ask the questions that have come to you. It may help you to write questions down and keep them in one place so that you can organize your inquiries. You can also call your health-care provider's office if you have questions between visits.

While online medical sites are a wonderful source of information, they are also very easy ways to misdiagnose yourself and cause needless worry. Use these sites for information and as a way of learning basic information, but leave diagnosis and treatment up to your health-care provider, who knows your specific situation.

You can also educate yourself by reading pregnancy books (like this one!) and Web sites about pregnancy. A wealth of information is available online and in bookstores. Many of your simple questions can be answered this way. You should never feel that your questions are too basic to bother your own health-care provider with. Whatever you want to know, she is there to discuss. Some women prefer to call the office and talk to a nurse. If this makes you more comfortable, do so.

Books and Web sites are useful because they can give you important background information and help you understand the terminology used when talking about pregnancy. They also let you know that you're not alone.

Lots of women have gone through what you are going through, and they've done so successfully.

Taking Control of Your Own Health Care

Health care for your pregnancy is for your body (and your baby's). When there are decisions to be made, you are the one who must be able to make them. Pregnancy is not a passive circumstance, and it is your right to make decisions and ask difficult questions.

Informed Consent

One of the basic rules of medical care (and also a legal right) is that the patient must give informed consent to any medical care. This means that as a patient, you have the right to first be informed about the treatment, its benefits, risks, and potential side effects. Once you have been informed, it is up to you to decide what will be happening to your body. Health-care providers can act without your consent in an emergency situation, but in all other cases, it is up to you to weigh the choices and decide what you will agree to. It is your choice not to accept treatment (except in some situations where the baby might be in danger).

Making Decisions

Lots of women feel that they have been trained not to ask questions, offer opinions, or stand up for themselves in medical situations. The good news is that pregnancy is something that happens gradually, so you will have time to arm yourself with questions, do some research, and come to your appointments prepared to make decisions.

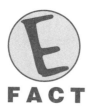

According to the U.S. Centers for Disease Control (CDC), 99 percent of U.S. births occur in hospitals, with the majority attended by doctors. Of the 1 percent that do not occur in hospitals, 65 percent are homebirths and 27 percent occur at birth centers.

There are a lot of decisions to make during pregnancy. Your health-care provider is there to offer information and offer recommendations, but in the end, you are the one who must make the decisions. It can be easy to just go along with what your health-care provider recommends. However, if you take the time to educate yourself and consciously make the decision yourself, you will feel more secure in the decision you have made and more in control of your body and your life.

Sometimes it can be frustrating to have your health-care provider present you with choices because you may feel you simply aren't equipped to make that kind of decision. First of all, remember that in most situations, these are not decisions that must be made on the spot. If you are deciding whether or not to have an amniocentesis, you have some time to make that choice. Secondly, make sure you ask enough questions. Ask everything you can think of, no matter how silly it may seem. Your health-care provider cannot make your choices for you, but he can make a recommendation. If your health-care provider seems to only be giving you the facts, and not a recommendation, feel free to ask for one. One thing you can do is say, "If it were you sitting here in my shoes, what would you choose to do?" If you still are unsure of what you want to do, ask to have some time to think about it. Talking these decisions over with your partner or with close friends or family is another way to work through the choices. If it helps, bring someone with you to your appointments so that he or she will also hear what your health-care provider is saying. Taking notes help you keep straight all of the information you've been given as well.

There are times when your health-care provider might seem to assume what your decision is without actually asking you to make a choice. If this happens, it's okay to slow things down, ask for more information, and take the time to make the decision yourself. Even if you ultimately make the decision that was being assumed, actively using your power to make that decision can make you feel you are in charge of your own body.

If a particularly controversial issue comes up, you should not hesitate to request a second opinion. Most competent physicians are not threatened by such requests because they are confident in their abilities and may actually welcome your discussing the issue with a second physician. Once the second opinion is rendered, both you and your doctor may feel more comfortable with your final decision.

How an Over-35 Pregnancy Is Monitored

You may be nervous or worried about the kind of care and monitoring an over-35 pregnancy requires, but you needn't be. You won't be under a microscope or treated as an oddity. The over-35 pregnancy is becoming more and more commonplace.

When you are over 35, your pregnancy is managed a little more closely than it would be for younger women. You may be aware that screening for Down syndrome is now offered to women of all ages; however it is highly recommended for older mothers. Your physician will discuss testing for this and other disorders with you and may recommend that you go to see a genetic counselor to help you understand your increased risk. While older mothers are at a higher risk of these kinds of problems, the odds are still overwhelming that you will have a healthy baby.

Because you are also at a higher risk for pregnancy complications, such as miscarriages, birth defects, preeclampsia (high blood pressure), gestational diabetes, placenta previa, and a low birth-weight babies, your health-care provider will be checking for these problems. Your health-care provider is there to catch problems early on and prevent complications. Your health-care provider does not expect to find problems simply because you are over 35 but is on the lookout for them with a careful eye. You should remember that risk in medical terms is relative. For example, though your physician may say that your risk of having a live baby born with Down syndrome is increased, the actual risk is only one in 356. Higher than what a younger woman would face, but the actual risk is not very high.

As an over-35 mother, you will not have more frequent prenatal appointments than other women unless you are experiencing problems. You can expect to be referred to a maternal-fetal medicine specialist for testing for things such as Down syndrome and spina bifida, but as long as you are having a normal pregnancy, you won't need to work with the specialist on a regular basis unless you specifically choose to.

Your health-care provider's job is to watch for any possible risks in your pregnancy and step in to manage them if they do appear. All pregnancies are about managing risk, and yours is no different. Your health-care provider is there to minimize risk and take action if risk does arise.

Your Birth Plan

A birth plan is an outline for how you want to have your labor and delivery managed. Birth plans are not binding documents, but they are a helpful way to think through the many options available to you and communicate that information to your health-care provider.

A birth plan is more of a way to start a conversation with your health-care provider than to put anything down in stone. It's important to weigh the options you have available and express your preferences to your health-care provider. At the same time, if something unexpected happens during childbirth, your health-care provider will do what is best for you and your baby. A birth plan allows you to have a conversation about your wishes and requests with your health-care provider in advance. In creating a birth plan, you may come across options you had not previously considered, so the process can be an educational one. You may wish to bring your birth plan with you to the hospital or birthing center.

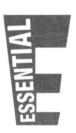

Create and save your own birth plan online using a birth plan tool at ✐*http://birthplan.com*. If you wish, you can print out copies for your doctor, send one to the hospital or birth center, give one to your coach, and bring one with you when you go in to deliver.

A birth plan can include the following:

- Place of birth (hospital, home, or birth center) and the criteria for moving from one location to another
- Length of time you will remain at home while in labor
- Birth positions
- Birth furniture and equipment (such as birth balls, birthing stools, or water-birth tub)
- Anesthesia and pain-relief options and preferences
- Comfort measures during labor (such as music, massage, lighting, or aromatherapy)

- Episiotomies
- Labor and birth coaches and assistants
- Length of stay in the hospital after the birth
- Consent for interns, students, or residents to observe your birth
- Use of film or photography
- Fetal monitoring methods (internal or external monitors, or sporadic monitoring)
- Intake of fluids and food during labor
- Wearing glasses or contacts during the birth
- Mobility during labor (whether you will have monitors attached, be able to walk around or shower)
- Rupture of membranes (natural rupture or planned rupture by your health-care provider)
- Labor augmentation (speeding up labor with drugs)
- Forceps or vacuum extraction
- A mirror to see the birth
- Contact with the baby immediately after birth (breastfeeding or skin-to-skin contact at delivery)
- Rooming-in (whether the baby will stay in your room or the nursery)
- Circumcision
- Cutting of the cord by the father or birth partner
- C-section

Birth plans can be written in several different ways. You can write it as a list of your preferences, explaining what your ideal birth would be and what alternatives you would consider should they become necessary. You can also write your birth plan as a solid list of decisions you have made that you are presenting to your health-care provider. No matter how you write your birth plan, it is something you are free to revise at any point during your pregnancy. Of course, you can change your mind about anything during labor and delivery as well.

Chapter 7

Risks

Every pregnant woman faces risks of some kind. Understanding what those risks are in a realistic way and understanding how to deal with them is important for all women. Women who are over 35 do have some elevated risks for pregnancy complications and birth defects, but a good health-care provider can help you manage, understand, and cope with whatever risks you are facing. The odds of having a healthy baby are strongly in your favor.

Calming Your Fears and Understanding Risks

It seems that when people talk about pregnancy for older moms, all they focus on is the risks. It is well known that older mothers have an increased risk of having a baby with Down syndrome (as discussed on page 78 and 94), and this seems to be the one fact that everyone knows and wants to talk about. While there is an increased risk for Down syndrome and other complications, the huge majority of women over 35 have a healthy baby and pregnancy.

When health-care professionals talk about risk, they are considering the possibility of something that could complicate your pregnancy. Risk is usually discussed as a percentage (a 5 percent risk of developing a certain complication means that five out of 100 women will experience it) or as a factor (one in 1,000 women experience this complication). It's important to keep in mind what these numbers mean. All they do is express how often this kind of thing happens.

It is also important to understand the concept of relative risk. In medicine, almost all risk is actually relative risk. For example, when there is a risk of lung cancer in cigarette smokers, this means the risk is significantly higher than it is among nonsmokers; nonsmokers still have a risk of lung cancer. Absolute risk is the actual risk you have of developing a problem. For example, if the risk of having a baby with a birth defect is one in 1,000 for one group of women and four in 1,000 for another group of woman, the relative risk is four times higher. It might sound impressive if someone told you that your risk was four times higher. Yet the actual risk is only four in 1,000, which in absolute terms is not very high. Though the risks of various pregnancy problems in older women are somewhat different, in actual terms, most of the actual risks are not high. Instead, they are higher relative to younger women.

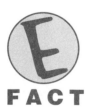

Women over 40 who give birth have a higher rate of left-handed babies. Their babies are also on average one inch shorter and three pounds lighter than babies of younger women.

Another important thing to keep in mind about risk factors is they are only factors; they are not solid predictors of what will happen in your pregnancy. Many, many women are at high risk for something, yet they never experience it.

Your health-care provider understands all of the risk factors that affect you and is there to watch for them, test for them, prevent them, and treat them if they occur. Let her do the worrying about risk factors. That's what you're paying her for! She's the professional who is trained to work with and assess risk. Your job is to focus on your baby and staying healthy. If you worried about everything that could possibly go wrong in your pregnancy, you would become quickly overwhelmed.

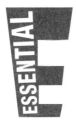

Down syndrome used to be a difficult diagnosis, but now babies born with Down syndrome can live to be fifty years old and can play sports, have jobs, go to school, and even get married, depending on their level of mental retardation. In addition, many people find that Down children are very special in the way they relate to the world and make other people feel.

It is true that as you age, your pregnancy risks do go up, but they don't skyrocket. No one is going to sit you down and tell you that this pregnancy thing was probably not a very good idea. It is too easy to get wrapped up in the slight increase of risk that you face. Your health-care providers will monitor your risks and cope with them. It's a wonderful thing that medical science is so advanced that it can predict an increase in problems as women get older because this allows health-care providers to be on the alert for these problems before they develop.

Reducing Risks

While there is nothing you can do about the risk factors that are calculated for your pregnancy based on your age, weight, and pre-existing conditions, there are many things you can do minimize risks in other ways.

Exercising and eating a healthy diet are two very important things you can do to keep your pregnancy on track. Follow your health-care provider's recommendations for weight gain in pregnancy. Too much weight gain can increase your risk of gestational diabetes, while not enough increases your risk of a low birth-weight baby. Take your prenatal vitamin regularly. If you have trouble swallowing it or keeping it down, ask your provider about alternatives, such as taking several children's chewable vitamins or some of the new chocolate vitamins you can purchase.

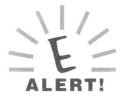

ALERT!

Despite the fact that alcohol and smoking have well-known risks to the fetus, the March of Dimes confirms that 13 percent of women report drinking during pregnancy, 3 percent report binge drinking, and 11 percent of women smoke during pregnancy. Avoiding alcohol and cigarettes are important steps you can take to protect the health of your baby.

Not smoking or drinking alcohol are two other very important steps you can take to protect your own health and that of your unborn child. Both habits increase the risk of a low birth-weight baby and preterm delivery. Smoking doubles the risk of placenta previa and increases the risk of miscarriage and stillbirth. Drinking increases the risk of birth defects. Avoiding alcohol and tobacco are significant ways to reduce your risks. Congenital anomalies (birth defects) occur in the first seven to nine weeks of the pregnancy. Many birth defects such as spina bifida and congenital heart disease occur by five weeks gestation. This is only one week past a missed period, at the point you might realize for the first time that you might be pregnant. Because of this, it is important to avoid alcohol, smoking, and other dangerous substances before you become pregnant.

Gestational Diabetes

Diabetes is a condition in which the body does not produce enough insulin (a chemical that allows the body to digest sugar or glucose), or is unable to use the insulin it has (insulin resistance). When this happens, sugar or glucose accumulates in the bloodstream and throughout the body, causing damage to internal organs, eyes, nerves, and blood vessels.

Gestational diabetes, which occurs during pregnancy, is a milder form of diabetes. Generally, the blood glucose levels in gestational diabetes are only mildly elevated compared to overt diabetes and do not cause a problem for the mother. These mildly elevated glucose levels can, however, affect the baby. These problems can cause the baby to be oversized, which can lead to delivery problems and an increased need for C-sections. Occasionally stillbirth can occur. The baby can have problems after birth such as hypoglycemia (low blood sugar) and jaundice. Childhood obesity and a predisposition to diabetes can also be a problem for the child.

Understanding Gestational Diabetes

Normal pregnancy requires the mother's body to make more insulin and for the insulin to work more effectively. When you develop gestational diabetes, you develop an increase in blood-glucose levels, usually after meals and at times when fasting. Gestational diabetes commonly develops in the second half of pregnancy (after twenty to twenty-four weeks).

Risks for Gestational Diabetes

Women over age 35 are twice as likely to develop gestational diabetes as younger women, who have a rate of about 3 to 5 percent. One study at Mount Sinai School of Medicine in New York City found that women over 40 were three times as likely to develop it. Gestational diabetes is on the rise among all women, with the U.S. Centers for Disease Control (CDC) reporting a 61 percent increase among all women between 1991 and 2001. The risk for gestational diabetes is elevated among people of Hispanic, Southeast Asian, Native American, and African American ethnicity.

Controlling Gestational Diabetes

If you do develop gestational diabetes, you will need to control your blood sugar with diet and exercise. You will need to test your blood sugar in the morning and one or two times throughout the day after meals. Most women can control gestational diabetes through diet and exercise, but a small number will need insulin injections or an oral medication called Glyburide.

Once you've had gestational diabetes, you have a 50 to 60 percent chance of developing adult onset or type 2 diabetes later in life. If you have had gestational diabetes, you should be screened annually for type 2 diabetes. This is important not only for your health but also to know if you develop type 2 diabetes prior to any future pregnancy.

If you do develop type 2 diabetes, it is important to have preconception care and achieve ideal blood glucose control prior to the pregnancy to avoid the risk of birth defects from high blood sugars. Fortunately, gestational diabetes alone is not generally associated with birth defects. If you have had gestational diabetes, your chance of developing the same condition in later pregnancies is high. You can significantly reduce that risk by weight loss, diet, and exercise prior to the pregnancy.

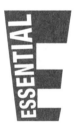

If you develop gestational diabetes, you will need to follow a special gestational diabetes diet called an American Diabetes Association (ADA) diet. This is not a caloric restriction diet, but one that carefully balances protein, carbohydrates and fat. If you have gestational diabetes, you should see a dietician to help you work out a diet you can follow.

Preeclampsia

Hypertension (high blood pressure) that develops after the twentieth week of pregnancy in a woman with no history of hypertension can either be gestational hypertension or preeclampsia. Distinguishing the two may be difficult. Preeclampsia is characterized by protein in the urine (proteinuria) and swelling (edema). Gestational hypertension is high blood pressure without these additional symptoms. Either condition may be problematic, but preeclampsia generally poses more of a danger to both mother and baby.

Understanding Preeclampsia

Preeclampsia can lead to central nervous system problems (including blurred vision, headaches, and confusion), stroke, and kidney failure. Preeclampsia left untreated can lead to eclampsia, a serious life-threatening condition that can cause seizures. Preeclampsia usually ends at delivery. Sometimes an especially serious variant of preeclampsia called HELLP syndrome can occur. It is characterized by involvement of the liver, red blood cells, and blood coagulation system. It can sometimes occur by itself, without preeclampsia.

Risks for Preeclampsia

Women over age 35 are twice as likely as younger women (whose risk is about 5 to 8 percent) to develop high blood pressure during pregnancy, one of the warning signs of preeclampsia. Women over 40 have a 60 percent chance of developing this. Risks are higher for women carrying multiples. Having a mother or sister who had preeclampsia increases your risk. Risk is also elevated if your baby's father's mother had preeclampsia when pregnant with him. This may be a genetic form of preeclampsia, in which the unborn baby inherits the trait and actually causes the preeclampsia.

Preeclampsia is more common in a first pregnancy. If you develop preeclampsia in one pregnancy, you are more likely to develop it in subsequent pregnancies. Interestingly, smoking decreases the risk of preeclampsia (although it is not recommended as prevention) and the use of barrier contraception, such as condoms or the diaphragm, in the year prior to the pregnancy increases the risk.

Controlling Preeclampsia

In women at very high risk for preeclampsia (such as those with existing renal disease or hypertension), low-dose aspirin was effective in preventing preeclampsia. However, the study did not focus only on women over age 35. Bed rest or medications can be prescribed to control preeclampsia. Although reducing salt intake is recommended for other cases of hypertension, it is not a recommendation for high blood pressure during pregnancy, so don't try this as a solution. If preeclampsia is becoming dangerous, induction of labor may be necessary, even if the baby is premature. Fortunately most preeclampsia occurs at the end of pregnancy, is mild, and can easily be managed by delivery.

Placenta Previa

Placenta previa is a condition in which the placenta, the pancake-shaped sac that provides nourishment to the baby, covers the opening of the cervix. Often this complication resolves itself, but in those situations when it does not, it is very dangerous.

Understanding Placenta Previa

Placenta previa is also sometimes called a low-lying placenta. Because the placenta is completely or partially blocking the opening of the cervix, labor will place pressure on the placenta, which can create a dangerous situation for the baby and also result in heavy bleeding.

Risks for Placenta Previa

The risk for placenta previa is about one in 200 (or .5 percent) for younger women. The risk increases with age, with women over 35 having a 1 percent risk. A University of California at Davis study found that women over age 40 had eight times the risk of younger women of developing this condition. You are at an increased risk if you are carrying multiples, have had previous C-sections, had placenta previa in a previous pregnancy, smoke, or have had uterine surgery.

Treatment for Placenta Previa

If your placenta previa is noticed in an ultrasound in your second trimester, you'll be sent for later ultrasounds to check on the location of the placenta. In 90 percent of cases, it moves up on its own. If it doesn't, you may be put on "pelvic rest," which means no intercourse or vaginal exams during your pregnancy and can also include an instruction to avoid heavy lifting. If your placenta previa persists, you will need to have a C-section. If you have ongoing bleeding and you are preterm, your baby may need some corticosteroids to improve his or her lung functioning for delivery prior to the due date.

Low Birth Weight

The term *low birth weight* traditionally was defined as a birth weight under 2500 grams, or 5 lbs. 8 oz. It was discovered that some of these babies were premature, some had suffered from intrauterine growth restriction, and some were constitutionally small (just small persons who are normal otherwise). Over time, the term has changed to mean a birth weight less than the tenth percentile for gestational age, which happens to be around 2500 grams for a term baby. Low birth weight is a concern because of the potential health risks to the baby.

Understanding Low Birth Weight

Babies that have low birth weight may be the result of preterm birth (as discussed on page 90) or intrauterine growth restriction, where they simply do not grow as large as they should due to problems with the placenta, birth defects, or problems with the mother's health. They also may just be small persons or constitutionally small. Distinguishing between these possibilities prenatally requires a great deal of skill and experience. Babies who are low birth weight due to prematurity or growth restriction are more likely to have problems as a newborn, including breathing problems, and to experience disabilities.

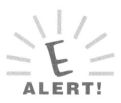

ALERT!

Signs of preterm labor include contractions every ten minutes, backache, bloody show, increased vaginal discharge, leaking fluid or blood, pelvic pressure, period-like cramps, and abdominal cramps. If you experience any of these, contact your health-care provider immediately.

Risks for Low Birth Weight

One in thirteen babies is born with low birth weight. Women over 35 are 20 to 40 percent more likely than younger women to have a low birth-weight baby, generally due either to prematurity or intrauterine growth restriction. Multiples are at a high risk of having low birth weight. African American babies have two times the rate of low birth weights as other babies.

Treatment for Low Birth Weight

Low birth weight can be predicted during pregnancy using ultrasound and fundal height (a measurement of the size of the uterus). If you are told your baby appears small, your health-care provider may encourage you to rest more often, avoid stress and strenuous exercise, and make sure you are taking in enough calories. Low birth-weight babies may need specialized care in a neonatal intensive care unit (NICU), where they are placed in heated beds, given feeding tubes, and monitored for breathing difficulties.

Preterm Birth

Preterm birth occurs when a baby is born before thirty-seven weeks of pregnancy. (A normal pregnancy lasts about forty weeks.) Many factors can contribute to this, including maternal age. Preterm birth is of great concern because these babies not only tend to have low birth weights, they are also not fully developed and are not yet ready to be born.

Risks

About 12 percent of U.S. babies are born preterm. The older a woman is, the higher her risk for preterm delivery. Women over 35 are 20 percent more likely to deliver preterm. Multiples almost always deliver preterm. Women who had previous preterm births are at a higher risk, as are women with abnormalities of the cervix or uterus or those who have pregnancies close together. Diabetes also increases your risk of preterm labor.

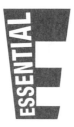

There may be a relationship between poor nutritional status, zinc and folic acid deficiency, and preterm labor, but a cause-and-effect relationship has not been established. Nonetheless, a good diet, as well as vitamin and folic acid supplements, may help reduce your risk. Recent studies have shown that in women with a prior history, weekly progesterone injections may help reduce the risk of preterm delivery.

Treatment

When a woman goes into preterm labor, her health-care provider will try to slow down or stop the labor by giving her a tocolytic, a medication designed to stop the contractions. The strategy when dealing with preterm labor is to delay it as much as possible. Sometimes it is possible to stop the labor, and in other cases physicians are able to delay the birth. Buying time is important. The primary concern is having enough time to administer drugs (corticosteroids) to improve the baby's lung function.

Babies born preterm may need help breathing and are often low birth weight. Very low birth-weight babies are at risk for brain bleeds. Other problems include heart problems, intestinal problems, vision problems, jaundice, apnea, and anemia. Despite this, the survival rates are quite good for preterm infants. Of those born at thirty-two to thirty-five weeks gestation, 98 percent survive. Babies born at less than twenty-eight weeks are at the highest risk for problems. Of those very preterm babies, 20 to 40 percent develop lasting disabilities. Infants born after thirty-four weeks, however, have excellent chances and only face possible learning or behavioral disabilities.

Multiples

Expecting not one but two or more babies at a time can bring incredible joy, but it is also something that can make your pregnancy more difficult. Often when talking about multiples, there is a distinction between twins and higher-order multiples. The more babies you are carrying, the higher the risks. The dramatic increase in multiples in recent years is due to the fact that more older women are having babies, and more people are using fertility treatments, both of which increase your chances of multiples.

The Facts about Multiples

Twins are the most common type of multiple, making up 95 percent of multiple births. While having twins is double the blessing, it can also mean more concerns. One third of twins are identical twins, formed from the same egg. Of these identical twins, 15 percent develop a serious condition called twin-to-twin transfusion syndrome, in which there is a connection between their blood vessels in the placenta. This can mean one twin can get greater blood flow than the other.

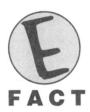

FACT

Twins make up 3 percent of all births in the United States, a number that is up 60 percent since the 1980s, according to the CDC. Age increases your risks of naturally conceiving twins. The likelihood of having twins peaks between ages 35 and 39.

African American women, women who are tall or large, and women who have had fraternal twins before are all at a higher risk for multiples. Additionally, the more pregnancies you have, the greater your risk for twins. Women over age 35 are more likely to have twins because their bodies produce more follicle-stimulating hormone (FSH), which causes more eggs to be released each month. In 2003, one out of eighteen births to women over 35 was multiples, compared to one out of thirty-three in women under 35.

Multiples are diagnosed by ultrasound and are usually spotted by the beginning of the second trimester. An abnormal result on the triple or quad screen blood test at sixteen weeks can also alert your health-care provider to multiples. If you have undergone fertility treatments, it is likely that your multiple pregnancy will be identified almost immediately. Additionally, your health-care provider may diagnose multiples by hearing two fetal heartbeats.

Complications with Multiples

The primary concern with multiples is preterm birth. When babies are born before thirty-seven weeks gestation, they are likely to have problems and face disabilities. Sixty percent of twins, 90 percent of triplets, and almost all higher order multiples are born preterm, and the length of the pregnancy on average decreases with each baby in the uterus: thirty-six weeks for twins, thirty-two weeks for triplets, thirty weeks for quadruplets, and twenty-nine weeks for quintuplets. Low birth weight is also common, not only because of the increased likelihood of preterm birth but also due to fetal growth restriction.

Multiples also increase the chances of the mother developing preeclampsia and gestational diabetes. Gaining enough weight early in the pregnancy is an important way to help keep your pregnancy healthy. Your health-care provider will want to see you more frequently throughout a multiple pregnancy. Mothers of multiples are also advised to cut back their activities by the twentieth or thirtieth week of pregnancy to reduce the risk of preterm labor. Placental abruption, where the placenta detaches from the uterine wall before delivery, is also common in multiple pregnancies. Miscarriage rates are also higher in multiple pregnancies.

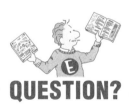

QUESTION?

If I undergo fertility treatments, will I have twins?
Fertility treatments greatly increase your risk of having multiples. Of women who give birth after undergoing fertility treatments, 56 percent have multiples. Reproductive specialists work hard to reduce the risk of multiples, but it is still a great concern.

Twin pregnancies can be delivered vaginally, although the chance of a C-section is increased. Other multiple pregnancies are always delivered by C-section. While all of this information might make you worry that your babies are at a greater risk, a National Institutes of Health study found that multiples of older moms were just as healthy as multiples of younger moms, so your age will not impact your babies' health.

Birth Defects

Birth defects are one of the things women worry about the most during pregnancy. While there is an increased risk for women who are over age 35 of delivering a baby with birth defects, these risks are not overwhelming. Many problems can be diagnosed during pregnancy using screening tests.

Chromosomal Abnormalities

Women over 35 years of age are at increased risk for having babies with chromosome problems. The primary point to remember is that while these risks are elevated, the odds are that you will have a healthy baby because only 3 percent of all babies are born with birth defects. Understanding these risks can help you make decisions about prenatal tests. (See Chapter 8.)

Chromosome problems are referred to as trisomies since they are associated with an extra chromosome of a specific pair. For example, a baby with Down syndrome has a total of forty-seven chromosomes instead of the usual forty-six; in this case, there are three number twenty-one chromosomes instead of two; hence, the term trisomy 21. Women over 35 are at risk for several trisomies, including trisomy 21, trisomy 31, and trisomy 18, as well as having babies with extra sex chromosomes. For example, instead of XX (girl) or XY (boy), one could have XXY, a special type of trisomy called Klinefelter's syndrome. Babies with trisomy 13 and 18 have a high mortality rate, with 90 percent having died from their disorder by one year of life; survivors are usually profoundly handicapped and often have multiple birth defects. More than half of the children with trisomies born to women over 35 will be Down syndrome babies.

Down Syndrome

Down syndrome is a chromosomal abnormality in the trisomy category, which means the child is born with three copies of a certain chromosome instead of the normal two. Children with this disorder are born with an extra twenty-first chromosome. This occurs in one out of every 733 births. The risk of Down syndrome increases with the mother's age. At age 30, the risk is one in 1,000. At age 35, the risk is one in 400. At age 40, the risk is one in 100. Interestingly, even though older moms have a higher risk of Down,

80 percent of Down babies are actually born to women under age 35; this is simply because there are more women having babies under 35. Once you have a baby with Down syndrome, your risk of having another is about one in 100.

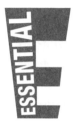

For information and support about Down syndrome, contact the National Down Syndrome Society (*www.ndss.org*; 800-221-4602).

Down syndrome is associated with a heart defect (50 percent of Down babies have this) and hearing and vision difficulties. These children have an identifiable look, with eyes that slant up and ears that fold over. They often have short necks, small noses, and small hands. Mental retardation can range from mild to serious.

Down syndrome, as well as trisomy 13 and 18, can be detected during pregnancy through a combination blood test and ultrasound, or through amniocentesis or chorionic villus sampling (CVS). See Chapter 8 for details about these tests. Recent studies have shown that women who have had a Down syndrome baby do not process folic acid normally, but studies into the causes of Down syndrome are ongoing.

Other Birth Defects

There are a wide range of birth defects, some of which are chromosomal and some of which are not. In general, older women are more at risk for all types of birth defects, but the increase in risk is small. Women ages 35 to 39 have an increased risk of 1.4 and women over 40 have an increased risk of 1.7 of having a baby with a congenital birth defect of any kind. Again, it is important to remember that this is relative risk; a younger woman has a risk of 1 percent (1 in 100) of having a baby with a birth defect. If you are 39, your risk is 1.4 times that, or 1.4 percent (14 in 1000). There is not an identifiable increase in any specific birth defect, though, just a slightly increased risk of any birth defect.

Most birth defects can be identified during pregnancy through screening methods available today (as discussed in Chapter 8). Some birth defects are minor. Some can be corrected after birth, while others are serious or life threatening.

Coping with a Diagnosis

Learning that your baby has or may have a birth defect can be devastating. It is often difficult to know what to do or where to turn. Get as much information as you can from your health-care provider and genetic counselor. Get details about how severe the defect is or is thought to be. Learn about the implications of the birth defect. Take some time to consider what you want to do. What kind of life would this child have? What would your life be like as the parent of a child in this situation? Are you able to cope with this defect? How would you cope? Contact the associations that are set up to support parents of babies with specific birth defects for information about support and education that is available to you. If you are considering terminating the pregnancy, ask questions about that procedure, your risk of having another baby with a similar defect, and your chances of conceiving again.

Chapter 8
Prenatal Testing

Prenatal testing is an important part of your pregnancy health care. Prenatal tests can reassure you that your baby is developing normally, that your pregnancy is progressing well, and that you remain in good health through the pregnancy. Prenatal tests are also important because they can isolate problems, such as birth defects, or determine when a baby is not thriving in the uterus. There are a wide variety of tests available. It is important to discuss available testing with your health-care provider to determine which tests are recommended for you.

How to Think about and Approach Testing

It can be easy to worry too much about prenatal testing and to make your entire pregnancy revolve around the tests and their results. Test results can be very helpful for you and your health-care provider if you approach them in the right way. One important thing to understand up front is that studies do not show that increased age is linked to an increased risk of miscarriage after an invasive test, such as amniocentesis.

Risk Versus Information

There are many prenatal tests that pose little if any risk to you or your baby. Blood tests, ultrasounds, physical exams, and so on provide your health-care provider with a lot of important information and are unlikely to cause you any problems. Other tests do carry some risks, particularly the risk of miscarriage when you are looking at amniocentesis or chorionic villus sampling.

Because some of these tests do carry a small but real risk of miscarriage, it is essential that you and your health-care provider talk frankly about what the real risk is to you and your baby. This chapter provides the national averages for risks; your health-care provider may be able to advise you further based on his own practice and on your particular pregnancy.

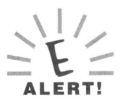

ALERT!

It can be easy to become nervous about prenatal testing. Reassure yourself by remembering that the odds of the test causing a problem for your pregnancy are quite small. The odds of an abnormal result are also quite small. In over 99 percent of cases, the test confirms the normality of the baby.

When deciding whether or not to have a test that a carries a risk, you need to evaluate whether the risk you face is worth the information you will get. Is there another way to get information that is as good? Would having the information change your plans for the pregnancy? Even if it would not change your decision about carrying the pregnancy to term, would it offer you information that would allow you to be prepared? Would it allow your health-care provider to take some precautions he might not otherwise?

Ultimately, the decision about whether or not to have a test is completely up to you. If you don't want the test, simply tell your provider this is the case. Before you make a decision, though, completely educate yourself about the following:

- How the test is done and what it feels like
- When in the pregnancy it is done
- How accurate it is
- What type of information it can provide

Dangers of a Test Compared to Risk

Another important factor you and your health-care provider need to consider is whether the risk of complications from the test itself is higher or lower than your risk for the abnormality being tested for. It is because of this comparison that age 35 is the age at which amniocentesis may be a reasonable option for some women. At this age, the risk of having a child with a chromosomal trisomy, such as Down syndrome, is higher than the risk of miscarrying from the test itself, so it is considered to be a risk worth taking. This merely indicates that from a risk-benefit point of view, the medical establishment considers it reasonable to offer the test. This does not mean that it should necessarily be done, particularly since there are other tests that are less invasive and that can provide good information with much less risk.

Dealing with Testing Fears

Pregnancy testing is fraught with a lot of anxiety. First, you may be nervous about the actual test procedure itself and any pain and discomfort you may experience. Next, you may dread the waiting period until you get results. And last but not least, you may be very nervous about what the results will show and what that will mean for you.

The best way to cope with test anxiety is first to gather as much information as you can. Ask specific questions about exactly how the test is performed, how long it takes, and what exactly it will feel like. It's your body and you're entitled to ask these questions, no matter how nervous or silly they may sound to you.

Be sure to follow your health-care provider's instructions before and after the test. If you are told to go home and put your feet up, be sure to do so. Your health-care provider is an expert about your test, and his or her instructions are important.

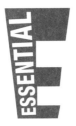

At your first prenatal visit, your health-care provider will do an internal and take a Pap smear to test for cervical cancer and STDs. In the final weeks of your pregnancy, your provider will do a cervical check to see if your cervix is opening, an indication that you are close to going into labor.

Ultrasounds

Almost all women have ultrasounds during pregnancy. This test allows your health-care provider to see an image of the baby using sound waves. Ultrasounds are recommended for all women over age 35.

Ultrasounds are used to determine or confirm due dates, look for multiple babies, check the baby's development, record heartbeats, measure the amount of amniotic fluid, and screen for abnormalities. Finding out the baby's sex can be one of the perks of this test, if you want the information. An ultrasound is performed by a health-care provider who moves a hand-held probe over the mother's uterus. Ultrasounds have no impact on the baby and are usually not uncomfortable, although you may need to have a full bladder for the test. If you have an ultrasound early in pregnancy or if you need one later in pregnancy to assess your cervix or to exclude a placenta previa or low-lying placenta, you will have a vaginal ultrasound. In this type of ultrasound, a probe is inserted into your vagina and gently moved, and an ultrasound image is generated that way. This is not painful, and you do not need to have a full bladder. It is also important to realize that this will not cause a miscarriage or any harm to your baby or the placenta.

A genetic ultrasound is a method of assessing for chromosome problems in women 35 and over. This is usually performed at sixteen to eighteen weeks. The ultrasound looks for markers and features of chromosome problems. If none is found, then the risk of trisomy 13, 18, or 21 is reduced by a certain percentage. The test cannot completely rule them out, but it can indicate the degree by which your risk is reduced. Some women use the genetic ultrasound to decide whether or not to have an amniocentesis. This method significantly reduces the need for amniocentesis. It is, however, very dependent on the skill and experience of the obstetrical sonographer.

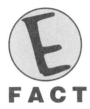

FACT

A study done by the Institute of Psychiatry at King's College London found that babies born to fathers who are over age 40 are six times more likely to have autism.

The first ultrasound is usually done around sixteen to twenty weeks (although some are done earlier to date a pregnancy, check for twins, or rule out an ectopic pregnancy). Later ultrasounds may be done during amniocentesis, to check positioning of the placenta, or to estimate birth weight. High-risk pregnancy may require more sophisticated ultrasound assessment using high-resolution ultrasound equipment and specialized testing such as fetal echocardiography (for a detailed evaluation of the baby's heart), or Doppler ultrasound (to measure velocity and flow of blood in fetal and uterine blood vessels). Generally a maternal-fetal medicine specialist performs such specialized surveillance.

Routine ultrasounds are usually performed by ultrasound technicians, and the results are then read and interpreted by a physician. This physician may be an obstetrician, radiologist, or maternal-fetal medicine specialist. Some obstetricians may hire an ultrasound technician to work full-time or part-time in their office so that the ultrasound may be done onsite. Generally, ultrasound results performed under the supervision of an obstetrician or maternal-fetal medicine specialist will be made available at the time of the scan. Results performed under the supervision of a radiologist generally are not shared with the mother at the time of the scan but are later reported to your obstetrical care provider, who then discusses the results with you.

It is important to remember that both the quality of the ultrasound imaging equipment and the skill and experience of the ultrasound technician and reading physician are extremely important. You will get the best results from a facility or practice with a lot of experience in obstetrical sonography. Sometimes, there may be a question of an ultrasound finding and a referral to a maternal-fetal medicine specialist or ultrasound unit will be recommended. If this happens, you should not panic, since most of these findings turn out to be nothing.

Blood Tests

Your health-care provider may order a variety of blood tests during your pregnancy. Blood tests are done with one needle prick, and one or more vials of blood are drawn. If you have difficulty having blood drawn, ask to lie down. Choose a focal point in the room or have someone with you who can distract and support you.

Initial Tests

The first time you see your health-care provider for a prenatal checkup, it is likely he will ask you to get some blood work done. These tests will give your provider information about your blood type, Rh factor (negative or positive blood type), anemia, syphilis, hepatitis B, HIV, immunity to things like measles and chicken pox, and cystic fibrosis. Sickle cell anemia testing is usually ordered for women of African or Mediterranean descent. Special tests may be ordered for women of certain cultural or ethnic backgrounds (such as Tay Sachs disease testing for Jewish women, and thalassemia testing for women of Mediterranean background). Testing may also be done for hepatitis C if the history warrants. Some obstetrical caretakers may screen for toxoplasmosis (parasitic infection carried by cats or caused by eating partially cooked meat or raw vegetables), or cytomegalovirus, though these are not routinely tested for in the United States. If you have a profession that puts you in contact with young children, such as teaching, your obstetrical caretaker may test your immunity to parvovirus, or Fifth's disease.

Gestational Diabetes

Screening for gestational diabetes is done using a blood test after you have fasted and then drunk a special glucose drink. About 15 percent of women test positive. Because this test does result in false positives, you'll be sent for a longer test in which several blood samples are drawn over a longer time period. Generally, 30 percent of the women sent for this test ultimately have gestational diabetes.

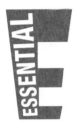

Urine tests are routinely performed at every prenatal visit to check the urine for protein (which can signal preeclampsia) and sugar (a possible indication of diabetes or gestational diabetes). You will either be asked to bring a sample with you in a sterile jar or provide the sample upon your arrival at the office.

The first round of testing takes place between twenty-four and twenty-eight weeks. If you are obese, had a previous baby that weighed over nine pounds, had previous adverse pregnancy outcome, have glucose in your urine, have had gestational diabetes or diabetes in the past, or have a strong family history of diabetes, you may be tested in the first or second trimester and will have a repeat test at twenty-four to twenty-eight weeks if the initial screen is negative. There is some debate about whether all women should be screened for gestational diabetes or only those with certain risk factors. However, there is general consensus that women over 25 and certainly over 35 should undergo routine screening. Many obstetrical caretakers will substitute other testing substrates, such as soda or candy, for the standard glucose testing solution that you drink for the test. As a general rule, only the standard testing solution is considered accurate for screening.

Other Blood Tests

Other blood tests done during pregnancy are used to screen for birth defects and abnormalities in the fetus. A first-trimester assessment is a blood test that screens for trisomy 21 (the chromosomal abnormality known as

Down syndrome) and trisomy 13 and 18 (other chromosomal abnormalities associated with advanced maternal age). Second-trimester testing includes AFP (alpha fetoprotein) and two additional hormones (triple screen) or three additional hormones (quad screen). The quad screen is currently considered the standard of care for second-trimester screening and is usually performed between fifteen and twenty weeks. It is best to screen as close to fifteen to sixteen weeks as possible so that timely testing can be performed if the test comes back positive. The quad screen assesses for trisomy 18 and trisomy 21, as well as spina bifida and other less common fetal abnormalities. A maternal serum AFP (MSAFP) may be performed alone, if the first trimester screen has already been performed and is negative, since the earlier screening tests cannot screen for spina bifida.

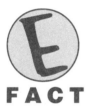

FACT

A quad screen does not screen for the chromosomal abnormality trisomy 13. This test is slightly less sensitive than a first-trimester blood test. Still, it is often used because in addition to trisomy 18 and 21, it can screen for spina bifida and other less-common birth defects.

If the quad test is positive, you may be offered the option of a genetic amniocentesis or a genetic ultrasound (as described on page 100–101). If the MSAFP is elevated, birth defects such as spina bifida can generally be detected by high-resolution sonography, and amniocentesis can usually be avoided.

It is important to understand the significance of a positive test result. These tests do not tell you that the baby does or does not have a chromosome problem. Instead, they give you an idea of the risk of specific chromosome problems, which may be high or low. A test only screens for the chromosome problems it was designed to detect (such as the sex chromosome trisomies described in Chapter 7). These tests detect a high percentage of babies with specific chromosome problems, such as Down syndrome, without resorting to invasive procedures. You should view a positive result only as an indication that you may need further testing. In the vast majority of cases, the baby is found to be normal.

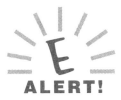
ALERT!

The AFP or quad screen detects Down syndrome 85 percent of the time and has a 7 percent false positive rate. In other words, 7 percent of women are told their fetus has a problem when in fact it does not.

It is important to discuss screening with your health-care provider prior to the test so that test results can be placed in perspective and you can decide if you want to undergo screening at all. Remember, when the screen is negative or it shows a relative low risk, then it is reassuring. However, a positive screen may cause considerable anxiety and theoretically could result in the loss of a normal baby if an invasive procedure is opted for. You should ask your physician about your actual age-related risk prior to screening. You may find that risk quite acceptable in absolute terms and may not wish to undergo screening.

Percutaneous Umbilical Blood Sampling (PUBS) or Umbilical Vein Sampling

This sampling (PUBS) tests blood from the umbilical cord. Although the long name makes this procedure sound awfully dire, it is a very simple procedure in which a physician uses ultrasound to guide a needle into the umbilical vein to sample the baby's chromosomes and test the baby for anemia. This test is very quick, with the same sensation as amniocentesis and offers quick results. There is a 5 percent adverse occurrence rate; adverse occurrence includes miscarriage or emergency delivery for a complication in a baby who is viable.

This test is recommended for women who have an inconclusive amnio result, are exposed to infectious diseases during pregnancy, or have babies who have Rh disease. The test is performed at eighteen to thirty-six weeks, and results are available within three days. This test does have a higher complication rate than standard amniocentesis and requires a skilled and experienced individual to perform the testing.

Combination Tests

Nuchal translucency screening (NTS) is a relatively new test that combines blood test results with special ultrasound results. It has been found to be highly accurate and an excellent noninvasive alternative to amniocentesis. NTS is generally recommended for all women (previously this was only recommended for women over age 35, but guidelines have now changed and this test is offered to all women) and is usually performed between the gestational age period of ten weeks, three days, and thirteen weeks, six days. Some women are referred for an amniocentesis or chorionic villus sampling based on the results, but many women decide not to have further testing after receiving reassuring results on this test.

The NTS uses a special ultrasound called a nuchal translucency test, in which space at the back of the baby's neck is measured. This measurement is used in conjunction with a triple or quad screen (and sometimes first-trimester blood work) to evaluate the risk for Down syndrome. When the ultrasound is done in conjunction with a second-trimester blood test, it identifies 95 percent of babies with Down syndrome. The test positive rate is approximately 5 percent; for every 100 women tested, five will have a positive result. The false positive rate is only slightly lower than the test positive rate, so most positive tests end up being false positives that ultimately show a normal baby. If the test is positive, you will be given the option of having a chorionic villus sampling or an amniocentesis later in the pregnancy, which will confirm or deny the presence of Down syndrome. If the baby has an increased nuchal translucency, but is found to have normal chromosomes, there may still be a risk of problems such as other genetic syndromes or congenital heart disease and further testing may be needed.

Some sonographers include assessment of the baby's nasal bone (some Down babies have poorly ossified nasal bones) as well as the baby's heart to detect tricuspid regurgitation (a leaky heart valve). The test screens for trisomy 13, 18, and 21 and is especially accurate for the detection of trisomy 21.

Some women 35 and over opt to go directly to chorionic villus sampling or genetic amniocentesis without having noninvasive screening first. Except in very rare cases, this will detect any chromosome problem. It has the advantage of certainty, but that comes with the disadvantage of the discomfort of an invasive procedure and a small risk of pregnancy loss. The risk of pregnancy loss may be particularly bothersome in the case of fertility patients who have tried so hard to become pregnant.

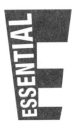

Fluorescent in-situ hybridization, or FISH for short, has largely replaced PUBS testing. This is a specific type of lab test that is done on a sample obtained during amniocentesis. This test can give you an answer in twenty-four to forty-eight hours on trisomy 13, 18, or 21.

There is some debate about combining first- and second-trimester testing. Sequential screening employs NTS first. If that is negative, then a second-trimester quad screen is performed. If either the NTS or the quad screen is positive, then invasive testing is offered. Integrated screening, the other option, involves both NTS and quad screening. After the quad screen result is known, both test results are integrated into a final risk. This differs from sequential screening in that the individual NTS and quad screen results are not individually interpreted. Instead, the results are put together after quad results return. The patient is not made aware of results until the integrated risk result is available. There is presently no consensus on which test method is better.

Fundal Height

Fundal height is a measurement of the size of your uterus. The height in centimeters should correspond to how many weeks along you are in your pregnancy.

Your health-care provider will take this measurement at every prenatal visit. He will find the top of your uterus and measure down, using a tape measure, to the top of the public bone. This measurement reassures you and your health-care provider that your baby is growing at the right rate. A smaller-than-normal measurement can indicate growth or development problems.

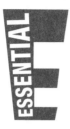

Fundal height measurements begin to lose accuracy after about thirty-six weeks of pregnancy because the baby settles down into the mother's pelvis, below the lowermost point of measurement.

Genetic Counseling

Genetic counseling is designed to help you sort through the diagnostic tests, screening tests, and possibilities available to you. A genetic counselor is a trained professional who works with pregnant women on a regular basis to evaluate these things.

Genetic counseling is recommended for all women over age 35, whether you plan to have screening and diagnostic tests or not. By examining family history as well as your ethnic background and age, the counselor will help you understand your risk factors for various disorders. The counselor will also explain how testing can help you examine your personal risk and assist you in interpreting test results.

Chorionic Villus Sampling (CVS)

Chorionic villus sampling (CVS) is a test that can detect Down syndrome and other chromosomal abnormalities, but it cannot detect neural tube defects. A thin tube is inserted through the vagina and cervix, or through the abdomen via a needle, to take a sample of the chorionic villi, wisps of tissue that attach the placenta to the wall of the uterus.

CVS is done at ten or eleven weeks of pregnancy (one month sooner than amniocentesis) and results are available within a week. CVS has a higher risk of miscarriage than amniocentesis (between .5 and 1 percent, according to the March of Dimes). It is considered to be more than 99 percent accurate. The test is recommended if a first-trimester screening indicates a risk of chromosomal problems, if a woman is at a higher risk for these kinds of abnormalities, or if waiting for an amniocentesis (which is done later in pregnancy) is not advised.

The advantage of this test is that it is more sensitive in detecting chromosome problems. It also offers information early in pregnancy, when termination is medically less difficult and the woman is likely to have more privacy in making the decision (since it is less obvious she is pregnant and a termination would not be as noticeable).

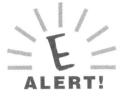

ALERT!

Since most twins are dizygotic (two fertilized eggs), the risk of at least one baby having Down syndrome or another chromosome problems is higher simply because there are two babies. Nuchal translucency screening and/or genetic ultrasound can be performed in twins. Some laboratories will adjust the first-trimester pregnancy hormone test or the quad screen for twins.

About 1 in 200 women have a miscarriage as a result of this test. In 1 to 2 percent of cases, a chromosome problem called mosaicism may be found, in which some cells have normal chromosomes and some don't. In this case, the chromosomal abnormality may be confined to the placenta and not be present in the baby. Generally an amniocentesis must be subsequently performed to confirm this.

Amniocentesis

Amniocentesis (commonly called amnio) is probably the most feared prenatal test and is the one most associated with pregnancies over age 35. An amniocentesis can provide accurate important information that is useful both to the mother and her health-care provider.

This test takes approximately a minute and uses a needle that is thinner than the one used to do a regular blood test. Your physician will use ultrasound to help guide the needle through your uterine wall and will take about one ounce of amniotic fluid to be tested. Some women feel cramping or a pinch during the procedure. This test diagnoses Down syndrome, spina bifida, and anencephaly conclusively (with 99 percent accuracy) and can also verify the baby's sex. Many women are concerned about the risk of miscarriage after an amnio. The pregnancy loss rate has traditionally been quoted as five in 1,000. However, it is has been shown that in experienced hands, using ultrasound guidance, that the risk is much less, probably in the range of one to three in 1,000. Physicians who are maternal-fetal medicine specialists and/or who do a large volume of genetic amniocentesis have much lower complication rates, which may approach one in 1,000. The take-home message is that more highly trained and experienced physicians have lower complication rates, so ask about your physician's experience level.

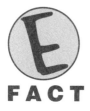

FACT

Male babies tend to be 4 percent heavier (averaging seven pounds, fourteen ounces) than female babies (which average seven pounds, nine ounces). Birth weight is also determined by birth order (later babies are heavier), maternal weight (heavier women have larger babies), duration of gestation (late babies are heavier), and ethnicity.

Amnio is recommended for women who have screening tests that indicate an increased risk of abnormality. If the risk of the abnormality is higher than the risk of miscarriage from the amnio, the test is recommended. This test is done at sixteen to eighteen weeks, with results taking anywhere from a few days to a few weeks. The long waiting period is often one of the most anxiety-producing aspects of this test.

Nonstress Test

A nonstress test is a third-trimester test that monitors the baby's movements. The test is done in a health-care provider's office. A belt is attached around the mother's belly for about half an hour to monitor uterine contractions and the baby's heart rate.

The baby's heart rate in response to movements she makes is monitored to determine if the baby is getting enough oxygen and to make sure the nervous system is responding. The test is said to be reactive if the baby's heart rate accelerated with movement and nonreactive if not. A nonreactive test may indicate a fetal sleep cycle rather than a problem. If the baby is asleep, a noise (acoustic stimulator) may be used to wake her up. Nonstress tests are ordered when there is a concern about fetal movement or if the pregnancy is high risk. Some practitioners routinely perform nonstress testing in the third trimester in women 35 or older. If the result is still nonreactive, a biophysical profile is recommended to study the baby's behavior by ultrasound.

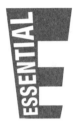

Between your thirty-fifth and thirty-seventh week of pregnancy, your health-care provider will do an internal exam and take a swab from the vagina and rectum to be tested for group B strep (GBS). 30 percent of women carry this bacteria, which can be passed to the baby during delivery and cause serious problems. If GBS is detected, you'll be given IV antibiotics during labor.

Chapter 9
Pregnancy Loss

While the odds are that you will have a happy and healthy pregnancy, it is important to understand that pregnancy losses do occur. The best thing you can do is stay positive about your pregnancy, do your best not to worry, and follow your health-care provider's recommendations.

Miscarriage

Miscarriage is medically defined as the spontaneous loss of a pregnancy before twenty weeks gestation. What you may not know about miscarriages is that they are far more common than most people think because many occur before a woman even realizes she is pregnant. Some studies indicate that 50 percent of all pregnancies end in miscarriage, some before implantation even occurs. Many early miscarriages are the result of genetic or chromosomal abnormalities.

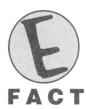

FACT

A 2000 Danish study found that about 9 percent of recognized pregnancies for women aged 20 to 24 ended in miscarriage. The risk rose to about 20 percent at age 35 to 39, and more than 50 percent by age 42.

Signs of a miscarriage include the following:

- Prolonged and heavy vaginal bleeding
- Cramping
- Sudden end of pregnancy symptoms such as breast tenderness, nausea, and fatigue

Types of Miscarriage

The medical term for a miscarriage is a *spontaneous abortion*. A miscarriage may occur and be complete, meaning that the pregnancy is completely lost and the cervix then closes. The medical term for this is a *complete abortion*. An incomplete miscarriage (medically termed an *incomplete abortion*) means a miscarriage has started but there is still tissue in the uterus, and the cervix is usually still open. If the cervix is open, but no tissue has been passed, a diagnosis of inevitable abortion is made, meaning that the pregnancy loss is inevitable. Because of the availability of early blood tests and ultrasounds, early miscarriages are frequently diagnosed prior to a woman experiencing any symptoms of miscarriage. Such pregnancies are termed *missed abortions*.

Sometimes, pregnancy loss after fourteen to sixteen weeks can be due to a special condition called *incompetent cervix* or *cervical insufficiency.* This occurs when the cervix dilates and thins painlessly, and the pregnancy literally "falls out" of the uterus.

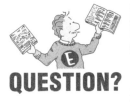

QUESTION?

If I had an abortion earlier in my life, does it affect my chances of having a healthy and successful pregnancy now?

In general, there is no evidence that a competently performed first-trimester abortion affects a woman's chances of having successful pregnancies later in her life. Late abortions (fourteen weeks and later) do have a small chance of adversely affecting future pregnancy outcome.

It is important to understand that more than half of women have bleeding during the first twelve weeks of pregnancy without having a miscarriage. By following the levels and trends of pregnancy hormones and using ultrasound, a physician can usually determine with reasonable accuracy the likelihood of a miscarriage for a woman who is experiencing bleeding. However, you should always check with your doctor if you experience any bleeding during pregnancy. Bleeding from a miscarriage can last seven to ten days.

Miscarriage Treatment

If a miscarriage is suspected, your doctor will order a blood test to test your pregnancy hormones and do an ultrasound to determine if the pregnancy is continuing in the uterus. Early miscarriages (under six to eight weeks gestation) usually do not require treatment. Usually, the woman will complete the miscarriage at home without medical intervention.

Miscarriages occurring between nine to twelve weeks may require medical or surgical intervention. Surgical intervention is usually in the form of dilatation and curettage (D&C) or suction curettage, in which the lining of the uterus is scraped and a special catheter attached to a vacuum is used to empty the uterus. Another option is medical curettage, in which drugs are given to the woman that cause uterine contractions, emptying the uterus. The procedure is generally begun in the hospital and completed by the woman at home. The medications are either given orally or as vaginal suppositories.

The decision as to whether medical intervention is required and the type needed (medical or surgical) is determined based on the gestational age of the pregnancy, the heaviness of bleeding, and the emotional state of the woman. Missed abortions are particularly difficult for many women emotionally. Many women have difficulty waiting for the miscarriage to start or taking medications to induce the pregnancy loss and opt for suction curettage. Medical curettage also has a small failure rate and surgical curettage may be required at a later point.

Curettage may also be recommended if your doctor wishes to send the miscarriage tissue for certain types of testing, such as chromosome analysis, to determine the possible cause of the miscarriage. Suction curettage may be performed in an examination room or in an operating room under anesthesia, depending on the circumstances. Miscarriages occurring after twelve to fourteen weeks gestation usually require formal medical evaluation and have a much higher chance for heavy bleeding and for requiring some form of medical intervention.

Once a miscarriage has been diagnosed by pregnancy hormones or ultrasound, or has already begun to happen, there is nothing that can be done to stop it. The one exception is an incompetent cervix. If this is diagnosed early enough, there is possibility of a cervical cerclage (a stitch placed around the cervix), which can prevent a miscarriage. For most miscarriages, you do not need to go to the hospital unless your doctor directs you to or if you cannot reach your doctor. Advil or Motrin, as well as a heating pad, is recommended for cramps.

If you pass tissue at home, it is important that you collect the tissue the best that you can and place it in some type of clean container or jar, preferably with a lid. This is important to confirm that you actually had a miscarriage and will help your doctor to determine if the miscarriage is complete. Sometimes in an ectopic or tubal pregnancy the woman may bleed and pass only the uterine lining. Without a tissue specimen, it can be very difficult to determine if the woman had a miscarriage or has a tubal pregnancy in progress.

Your doctor may follow up after the miscarriage with testing to try to determine if there was a cause. The amount and types of tests vary with the gestational age of the miscarriage, your age, or how many previous miscarriages you have had. Because you are over 35 years old, you should request that your doctor send the miscarriage tissue for chromosome testing. If a chromosome abnormality is found, other underlying causes of miscarriage are excluded, saving you from additional testing. If you have repeat miscarriages, you may be referred to a specialist. If the fetus was recovered during the miscarriage (usually only in a late miscarriage), your doctor may wish to do testing on the remains. Your physician will most likely recommend that you wait one cycle before trying to conceive again.

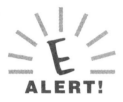

ALERT!

Call your doctor immediately if you experience vaginal bleeding, abdominal pain or cramping, persistent back pain, weakness, dizziness, or urinary pain or burning at any time during pregnancy.

The most important thing to understand about miscarriage is that it is not the woman's fault. There is nothing a woman can do to prevent or stop a miscarriage from happening. Most are nature's way of handling an abnormality. This, however, does not mean that the miscarriage is not a loss and is not important. You should grieve for your lost baby and give yourself time to cope with it. It also does not mean that you are somehow defective as a woman and that you won't be able to have a successful pregnancy in the future.

Well-meaning friends and family often say things that aren't exactly helpful, such as "It's nature's way of correcting a mistake" or "It's better than having a child with a deformity" or "You'll have another one." These people think they are helping, but they may not be. Take the time you need to mourn the loss you have suffered, and don't let what people say get to you.

Ectopic Pregnancy

An ectopic pregnancy occurs when the fertilized egg implants in the fallopian tubes instead of the uterus. (Though this is the most common locale, the fertilized egg can also implant in the ovary, abdomen, or cervix.) A pregnancy that implants in one of these areas cannot grow to term. The uterus is the only place a pregnancy can grow properly. If an ectopic pregnancy continues, it will cause the tube to burst. This can cause bleeding and endanger the mother's life, which is why an ectopic pregnancy is of great concern.

Causes of Ectopic Pregnancies

The risk of ectopic pregnancy increases as a woman ages, and women over age 35 have a risk that is three to four times higher than that of younger women. Some physicians believe that as a woman ages, the myoelectrical activity (the nerve activity that stimulates the fine hairs, called cilia, in the tubes to gently move the egg along) in her tubes decreases. When this movement slows down, it makes it more likely a fertilized egg won't be moved quickly enough to the uterus and will instead implant in the tube itself.

Ectopic pregnancies also often occur if there is blockage or inflammation in the tubes (more likely as a woman ages), making it difficult for the egg to travel through them. The risk of ectopic pregnancy is highest in women who have had PID (pelvic inflammatory disease), infertility, luteal phase defect, previous ectopic pregnancies, pelvic surgery, surgery involving a fallopian tube, or who have taken fertility drugs. An ectopic pregnancy is four times more likely when fertility drugs are used.

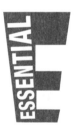

A study in the *British Medical Journal* found that by the time women reach age 35, one in five pregnancies ends in miscarriage, stillbirth, or ectopic pregnancy. While this number might seem high, remember that four out of five pregnancies have happy endings.

If a woman's mother took the drug diethylstilbestrol (DES, used for miscarriage prevention up until 1971) when pregnant with her this is another risk factor. Congenital malformations of the uterus, fibroids near the tubal insertion into the uterus, hormonal fluctuations found in older women, smoking, and vaginal douching have also been indicated as possible risk factors for ectopic pregnancies. A chromosomally abnormal embryo is also more likely to implant in the tubes than in the uterus.

If a woman becomes pregnant while she has an IUD, it is more likely the pregnancy will implant in the tubes. Progesterone IUDs and progesterone-only contraceptive pills may increase the risk of ectopic pregnancies, since the progesterone affects tubal functioning.

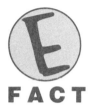

FACT

Of women who have had an ectopic pregnancy, 30 percent have difficulty getting pregnant again, but 70 percent do not and are able to have successful pregnancies. If you go on to get pregnant again after an ectopic pregnancy, you may be very nervous about having another ectopic pregnancy, but an early ultrasound can ease your worries.

Stopping smoking and removing a progesterone IUD can decrease the risk of ectopic pregnancy. Other than this, though, there is nothing you can do to prevent ectopic pregnancy. If you are at high risk, you will be monitored more closely at the beginning of your pregnancy. If you are seeing a fertility specialist, it is likely your pregnancy will be monitored by ultrasound from the very beginning to rule out an ectopic pregnancy.

Signs of an Ectopic Pregnancy

An ectopic pregnancy can be difficult to identify because the beginning symptoms are the same as for a normal pregnancy (missed period, nausea, painful breasts). The biggest red flag for an ectopic pregnancy is abdominal pain, which is not normal for a healthy pregnancy. The pain is often focused on one side, but it can occur anywhere in the abdomen or even up to the shoulders if blood builds up.

Other symptoms include the following:

- Dizziness
- Vaginal spotting or bleeding
- Fainting
- Low blood pressure
- Pain in the lower back or shoulder

If you experience any of these symptoms, you need to contact your physician immediately, but don't panic. More often than not, even with the symptoms listed above, a normal pregnancy is occurring. All of the symptoms above can occur in a normal pregnancy. Frequently, the ovary from which you ovulated (the corpus luteum) can enlarge, become tender and even bleed a bit. However, you should always report any symptoms to a physician.

If an ectopic pregnancy is suspected, your physician will do a pelvic exam and ultrasound to determine if there is implantation in the tubes. Your pregnancy hormones may be tested; a lower-than-normal level can also confirm an ectopic pregnancy.

If you already have risk factors for an ectopic pregnancy, it is even more important to seek immediate medical attention. In patients known to be at high risk for an ectopic pregnancy, the physician will generally not wait for symptoms but will follow HCG levels and do ultrasounds.

Treatment

An ectopic pregnancy cannot be moved to the uterus, as there is no way to move the embryo once it is implanted, nor can it be removed and frozen. Only unimplanted embryos created during fertility procedures can be cryopreserved in this way. If the mother's HCG level (pregnancy hormone) is low, she has no symptoms, and the HCG levels continue to decline, no treatment may be necessary. A large percentage of ectopic pregnancies end on their own without treatment.

If the mother has no symptoms and is stable, but the size of the pregnancy, presence of a live embryo, and high HCG levels are of concern, medical treatment with methotrexate injection to medically end the pregnancy and have the mother's body expel it is an option.

In other cases, surgery is necessary to remove the implanted fertilized egg. In many cases, this can be done by laparoscopy, a minimally invasive procedure done as an outpatient procedure. Often the ectopic pregnancy can be removed from the tube, leaving the tube intact. However, this is not always possible. In most cases, the tubes remain healthy after an ectopic pregnancy, but in some cases, scarring may result and the tube might not be functional again.

While there is no chance of ectopic pregnancy surviving, that does not mean that the end of the pregnancy is not a loss. Losing an ectopic pregnancy is just as devastating as any other type of pregnancy loss, and you must take time to grieve for it. And because a woman who experiences an ectopic pregnancy may have surgery, the physical recovery period may be longer than with a miscarriage. The stress involved in an ectopic pregnancy is also great. It is a dangerous condition and one that must be treated immediately, so in addition to the grief over losing a pregnancy, there is also emotional recovery from the stress and urgency of the situation.

It is important to remember that if you have had a previous ectopic pregnancy, your chances of having another ectopic pregnancy increase significantly. This makes it important to see your doctor very early in any subsequent pregnancies.

Stillbirth

A stillbirth is the death of a baby in the womb in the second half of pregnancy. The medical term for stillbirth is *fetal death*. In the United States, a fetal death is defined as the death of a fetus at twenty weeks gestation or more, and a late fetal death is at twenty-eight weeks gestation or more.

A large study published in the *New England Journal of Medicine* showed that the overall fetal death rate in the United States was 3.2 for every 1,000 live births. For women between the ages of 35 and 39, the rate was six for every 1,000 live births; for women over 40, the rate was ten for every 1,000 live births. Age itself is a risk factor for fetal death. However, conditions such as hypertension, diabetes, multiple gestation, placental separation, and placenta abruption occur more frequently in women over 35 and account for much of the fetal death rate in this age group.

For about half of all stillbirths, no medical reason can be determined. In other cases, there are problems with the placenta, umbilical cord, mother's health, or birth defects. It is important to understand that a stillbirth is not the mother's fault. There is nothing she can do to prevent it, other than getting good prenatal care and following her doctor's recommendations. Also keep in mind that the vast majority of women over 35 will not experience a stillbirth.

The biggest sign or symptom of a stillbirth is a decrease or lack of fetal movement in the uterus. Vaginal bleeding may be another indication there is a problem. If you experience either of these symptoms, you should call your doctor immediately. Your physician will check for a heartbeat using a handheld Doppler and may perform an ultrasound.

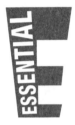

For support and information about stillbirth, contact the National Still-birth Society at *www.stillnomore.org*. Joining a support group can be very helpful, because you will be able to talk to other parents who have experienced the same difficult situation you have.

If a baby dies in the uterus, the mother will still need to go through labor and delivery (which may happen naturally or need to be induced) to expel the remains. This can be difficult and traumatic. Whether the pregnancy ends early in stillbirth or goes to term and has the terrible outcome of still-birth, parents are encouraged to hold the baby and spend time with him. You can also ask for mementos such as ID bracelets and photos. Your physician will perform a series of blood tests and send the placenta for evaluation. She may also wish to perform an autopsy to determine the cause of the stillbirth, but that decision is up to the parents. Deciding on an autopsy can be difficult at time of loss. However, if a cause can be found, it may provide closure as well as emotional relief. It may also help to prevent a similar occurrence in your next pregnancy. If you face stillbirth, do not be afraid to ask for help, such as a grief counselor.

If a woman has a stillbirth, it does not seem to increase her odds of a future stillbirth. While younger women might be encouraged to wait several months before trying to conceive again, women over 35 are usually encouraged to attempt conception six to eight weeks afterward.

Multifetal Pregnancy Reduction

Sometimes also called selective reduction, multifetal pregnancy reduction is a medical procedure in which a higher-order multiple pregnancy (triplets or higher) is reduced to twins or a singleton pregnancy. A recommendation for this procedure is made because the risks increase substantially when a woman carries three or more babies. It is also much more likely the pregnancy will end early—over 90 percent of triplets and virtually all higher number pregnancies end in preterm labor—and that the surviving babies will have disabilities.

The decision to undergo this procedure must be done early in pregnancy, usually before twelve weeks. The procedure involves injecting (using ultrasound as guidance) potassium chloride into one or more of the fetuses, stopping the heartbeat.

The procedure is generally performed between eleven and twelve weeks gestation. Some physicians recommend waiting as long as possible before reducing the pregnancy. This is because many multiple pregnancies experience what is called a vanished fetus, in which one or more of the fetuses are naturally reabsorbed by the mother's body and do not continue the pregnancy.

Multifetal reduction is generally considered safe and necessary in many cases. However, one of the concerns with the procedure is that there is a 6- to 8 percent chance of losing the other fetuses. The risk increases with the number of fetuses in the pregnancy.

Deciding to do a reduction is very difficult. Most often, the woman has undergone fertility treatments and worked very hard to get pregnant. The thought of reducing a pregnancy that was so difficult to achieve can be painful. It can be difficult to consider what the lost fetuses might have become. However, this procedure gives the remaining fetuses a greater chance at survival and good health. Should you find yourself in this position, talk with your doctor about the recommendation, procedure, and outlook. Each woman must weigh the risks and benefits of the procedure herself and come to her own decision.

Pregnancy Termination

The choice to end a pregnancy is one that is up to the woman involved. There are three options available. Plan B is a pill a woman can take within seventy-two hours of unprotected sex. At this point, she has no way to tell whether she is pregnant. The pill prevents the fertilized egg from implanting in the uterus.

Once a pregnancy has been confirmed, there are two options for termination. A medical abortion is done by taking two doses of medication that causes the end of the pregnancy. A surgical abortion is usually done by vacuum aspiration. If you need information on where to get help ending a pregnancy, contact Planned Parenthood (online at *www.plannedparenthood.com*) for information about local offices.

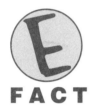

FACT

According to the CDC, about 24 percent of all U.S. pregnancies end in abortion. Women aged 40 to 44 make up only .2 percent of those who have abortions.

While a pregnancy termination is done by choice, it is still a difficult decision and is a loss. Making the decision can be painful. If you make this choice, give yourself time to heal and recover.

Recovering from Loss

The end of a pregnancy is a painful time. No matter how or when the fetus was lost, the mother is hit with the double whammy of physical symptoms as well as emotional ones. It is common to feel regret, relief, anger, sadness, grief, anxiousness, guilt, confusion, and more. Some women become certain that the end of the pregnancy was their fault and that there was something they could have done to prevent it. When a miscarriage or stillbirth is experienced, there is nothing the woman could have done.

Blaming yourself and agonizing over what you could have or should have done differently isn't helpful. Pregnancy losses do not occur because of any negative or ambivalent feelings the woman might have had about the pregnancy. In fact, it is quite common to have good as well as bad feelings about a pregnancy, even if it was one that was long awaited or carefully planned.

Many women find that one of the hardest parts of losing a pregnancy is that the loss is not acknowledged in the same way as the death of another loved one. The parents feel as attached to the lost child as they would to anyone they lost. Since many women do not share news of their pregnancy before the end of the first trimester, a pregnancy is often lost before many people are told about it. In those cases, no one is even aware of the loss, or people may find out about the loss without ever having known about the pregnancy.

Another reason pregnancy loss is difficult is because with miscarriage in particular, there often is no medical intervention at all. A woman is often encouraged to stay home and care for herself there. It may feel like the medical profession does not care or have much interest in the loss. Unfortunately there is nothing a doctor can do to stop a miscarriage, and so the loss is something a woman must handle on her own with the support of family and friends.

It takes time to recover from a pregnancy loss. Six months after a miscarriage, 50 percent of women are clinically depressed. If you experience a pregnancy loss and are experiencing severe depression symptoms, talk to your doctor. Depression is something that can be managed very well with medication and therapy.

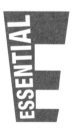

For support, memorials, and information about getting through a pregnancy loss, visit some of these Web sites: *www.pregnancyloss.com*, *www .nationalshareoffice.com*, *www.bornangels.com*, and *www.october15th .com*. Pregnancy and Infant Loss Remembrance Day occurs on October 15 of each year.

One way to cope with the loss is by talking about it. Even if you haven't told people about your pregnancy, you can share your loss with them. Because miscarriages are so common, you will probably find that many friends and relatives have experienced them. Another way to manage is to find a way to commemorate the lost child. Some people post on pregnancy loss Web sites, create their own Web sites, or create small memorials at home.

While the sharpness of the loss recedes, a lost child is something you never forget. Many women however, are able to move forward and achieve successful pregnancies after a loss.

Trying Again

After losing a pregnancy, many women wish to try to become pregnant again. Some women feel they can't or don't want to try again; that is a perfectly normal reaction as well. Some women feel they want to try again as soon as possible, while others feel they need to wait until they are ready. Be sure to discuss with your physician how long you physically should wait, but decide on your own how long you need emotionally. It is important to keep in mind your age and difficulty you may have had conceiving in the past when weighing the decision of how long you wish to wait.

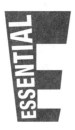

Recurrent pregnancy loss in women over 35 is the loss of two or more pregnancies before twenty weeks. Less than 5 percent of all women experience the loss of two consecutive pregnancies, and 1 percent will experience the loss of three or more. Of women who experience recurrent loss, 60 to 70 percent go on to have a successful pregnancy without treatment.

Many women do not feel they have completely emotionally healed from a pregnancy loss until their due date passes. Holidays may be very difficult after a pregnancy loss, and it is important to celebrate the people in your life that love you and support you at this time.

Chapter 10

Preparing Your Family for a Baby

Getting ready for a baby entails more than going to your prenatal checkups, taking your vitamin, and shopping for a layette. A baby is a major life change for everyone in your household. There are many things you can do to prepare yourself at work, at home, and financially.

Work Leaves and Career Changes

No matter what your career, having a baby has some impact on you because you need to take at least some time off from work. How much time you want or need is an individual choice. Some women make plans, but then find that once the baby comes, their feelings have changed. They either want more time off or feel they are ready to return to work sooner than they thought. Nothing you decide is written in stone. Before you can make maternity leave plans, you must first find out your options.

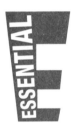

If your doctor advises you to stop working at the end of your pregnancy, you can use your sick leave time and may also be able to continue to receive payments under your employer's or state's disability leave program. To be covered, you'll need a note from your doctor.

Maternity Leave

Your company may have a maternity leave policy that allows you to take a certain amount of paid leave after the birth of a child. (Your partner's employer may also have a paternity leave policy, offering him paid time off, so be sure to check into that.) In California, Hawaii, New Jersey, New York, and Rhode Island, state disability leave programs pay a new mother a percentage of her pay for a certain number of weeks after having a baby.

Family Leave

The Family and Medical Leave Act (FMLA) is a federal law that allows people to take unpaid leave for the birth or adoption of a child, while keeping their job available for them when they return. This law applies to public agencies and private employers with fifty or more employees. To qualify, you must have worked twelve months and at least 1,250 hours in those twelve months. Note this is an unpaid leave, so you will need to plan for the financial impact.

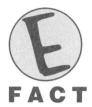

FMLA also allows work leave for an illness you have or to care for an ill family member. You or your spouse can therefore use it during your pregnancy as well as after the birth.

Under the law, you can take up to twelve weeks of unpaid leave in a twelve-month period. No medical documentation is needed to qualify when you have a baby. You can take the time as one big block, or you can use it to cut back your hours. Your spouse can also take this type of leave from his employer if he meets the requirements. If you both work for the same employer, you're only entitled to twelve weeks total between the two of you.

While you're on FMLA leave, your employer must keep your health benefits in place (although you may be required to pick up the premiums during your leave). When you return, you must be restored to your original job or an equivalent job with equivalent pay. Your employer can't penalize you for taking the leave or have it affect your benefits.

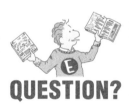

How do I apply for FMLA leave?
You must give your employer thirty days' notice of a foreseeable leave, so notify her about a month or six weeks prior to your due date. If you are suddenly put on bed rest or deliver early, notify your employer as soon as you can.

You will be required to take sick or vacation leave first, before FMLA time. Your state may also have a family-leave law that will apply to you, which you may be required to use first. It also makes sense to use your employer maternity leave or disability leave first, since those are paid leaves.

Planning for Work after the Baby

If you will be returning to work after the baby comes, you will want to start considering your options now so you can lay the groundwork with your employer. You may wish to return to your regular schedule as soon as possible, which can be a great way to get yourself back on track. If this is the case, let your employer know, because he or she might assume you will be taking a lengthy leave. On the other hand, you might be considering making some adjustments at work to allow you more time at home.

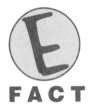

FACT

For help and support as you face life as a working mother, contact 9 to 5, National Association of Working Women (*www.9to5.org*; 800-522-0925).

Reducing your hours or going part time for a while after the baby arrives is one option to consider. Flex-time is another option that allows you to work the same number of hours but in more convenient configurations, such as four ten-hour days or starting an eight-hour shift later in the day, instead of a traditional schedule.

Job-sharing is another alternative to consider. You and another employee share one full-time position and arrange to split regular business hours between you. If you're interested in these options, find out if they have been used successfully by other employees in your company and think about how they might fit into your life. When considering any of these nontraditional work arrangements, you'll need to get approval from your employer.

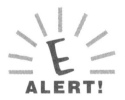

ALERT!

When you propose flex-time or job-sharing to your employer, put together a formal proposal that shows how the arrangement will benefit the company and that it will not cost the company more. Be sure to reference other employees in the company who have made this type of arrangement work.

Many women are concerned about being put on the mommy track after having children. It is true that choosing part-time work, flex-time, or job-sharing is likely to slow down your career. It is entirely possible to have a baby and maintain your momentum at work if you make it clear to your employer that your job is a priority in your life.

Other Children

If you have other children, you will want to help them get ready for the arrival of a new sibling. Give your child age-appropriate information about the pregnancy and birth, and try to involve him in the preparations for the new baby. Giving a child the responsibility for choosing a new toy or a mobile for the baby will help him feel important and connected.

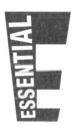

The Lee Middleton Company (*www.leemiddleton.com*) makes life-size, life-like newborn dolls that are close to the same size and weight as real newborns. You can order online, or you can take your child to a local store where they have a Lee Middleton "newborn nursery" section with dolls displayed in clear bassinets and staff dressed in scrubs.

A newborn doll may help young children get used to the size and shape of a newborn. Books about new babies can also help your child understand what is about to happen. Just talking to your child and answering all of her questions is very important at this stage.

Lifestyle Changes

Getting ready for a baby to join the family means making some adjustments to your life. In no way does this mean you have to become frumpy, boring, and out of touch. You can still have friends, do activities, look good, and live a full life with a baby, but it takes some adjustment. The first thing you should do is lower your expectations of yourself. No one is a perfect mother, no matter how hard she tries, how much help she has, or how well she copes. And no one spits out a baby and moves on with life as if it never happened. A baby creates change. You will need to adjust to your new life, and it will take time. You need to alter your mindset so that you are patient with yourself, your family members, and with the baby as well.

This is a good time to reassess some of the things in your life. If you have a gym membership now that you rarely use, you might find that after the baby comes you'll have even less time. Alternately, you might find that working out to get your body back in shape becomes a priority. If you have season tickets to a local sports team or theater, you might find that is something you will want to cut out once the baby comes, or you might feel that keeping some scheduled adult time is very important to you. A baby might also mean you will need to reconsider your living arrangements. A move might be in order to gain some space, or you might find you want to move to a more suburban area.

Classes

You're probably planning to take a childbirth preparation class to help you get ready for the birth of your baby. All childbirth classes are not made equal. Some classes focus on a specific technique, which can be great if that is the technique for you, but a class that offers a look at a variety of techniques may be more helpful. Most classes run four or six weeks, with one meeting per week, but many classes also offer a full weekend seminar, some at resorts or spas so you can have a complete "babymoon." Check with your insurance company about discounts on childbirth, baby care, sibling, and infant CPR classes. Some classes may even be free through your plan.

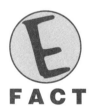

FACT

The Lamaze method is the best-known childbirth method. It teaches breathing and relaxation techniques and encourages a mother to rely on a labor partner for support, assistance, and massage. The goal of the method is natural childbirth.

If you have other children, you will want to consider sibling classes for them. These classes are held at the hospital where you plan to give birth (if you are planning on a hospital birth). An instructor talks to the children about how to care for newborns and what to expect when the baby arrives. The highlight of the class is a visit to the newborn nursery.

There are a variety of other classes that are probably available to you. Breastfeeding classes can help you learn techniques, troubleshooting, self-care, and comfort measures. Infant care classes teach things such as diapering, bathing, sleep techniques, and more. Infant CPR classes train parents to save their child's life in case of choking.

Planning for the Future

Now that you will be a parent, you may feel some of the responsibility beginning to weigh on you. Raising a child does mean keeping an eye on the future while enjoying today. Suddenly you're not just responsible for your own future; you have a family to plan for.

Refocusing Your Goals

Until you became pregnant, most of your goals were personal ones. You and your partner probably had some mutual goals about your life together, but you still remained separate individuals with separate careers, incomes, friends, hobbies, and more. Now that you are having a child, you still have your separate goals, but much of what you're dreaming about is family goals.

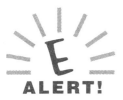

If you had your last baby by C-section and a vaginal birth is a possibility this time, you should take a VBAC (vaginal birth after cesarean) class to learn techniques to optimize your chances for a vaginal birth this time.

It can feel odd to suddenly go from individual goals to collective goals. Instead of being a woman with a partner, you're suddenly going to be part of a family. You may feel like you are becoming less of an individual. You can keep your own personal goals alive while embracing the goals you are creating for your family.

It may be helpful to make a list of goals you have for yourself personally as well as goals you have for your family. You may find that many of them are compatible—or that they can be, with a little work.

Choosing a Course for the Future

A lot of the time, it may seem like the future just happens to you. You have so little control in so many areas of your life—what job you will be offered, if you will find a life partner, where you will find an apartment, your health, and so on. Having a child is something that requires planning and careful thought. When you're having a baby, you suddenly see that the future is something you must direct. When you know you are going to be a mother, you suddenly must plan not only for your future but for your baby's as well. Suddenly, making mistakes and going with the flow may not seem as appealing as before.

While you may have a greater sense of purpose now, you can't carry the weight of the world on your shoulders. You can only work with what you have and the choices that are before you. You can, however, think about what direction you want your family to grow toward. For example, if you currently live in an urban environment, you might be thinking that a move to a suburban area is more in line with your family vision. A high-stress career may not fit well with your plans to spend a lot of time with your child. There are many things to think about, and you have a lot of time to work through them. Your child has eighteen years to grow up, and you have plenty of time to shape and mold your family.

Emergency Preparedness

While no one wants to consider the fact that a natural or man-made disaster could strike, it's a good idea to discuss a plan with your partner should one occur. This is particularly important during pregnancy, when you may feel particularly vulnerable or less mobile. You'll also want to have a plan in place for once your baby arrives. Disaster plans include the following:

- Preparing emergency supplies of food and water
- Designating a meeting place and a backup
- Noting the nearest hospital and a backup

- Having a plan to access cash if necessary
- Designating an out-of-state contact person you can use to relay messages
- Having medical records and necessary medications on hand
- Completing authorization for close family members to pick your child up from child care or to obtain medical care for the baby in your absence

Preparing Your Home

Getting ready for a baby can be a big logistical adjustment. Your home will now need to accommodate a baby, a whole new person who comes with a whole lot of stuff. Your baby will impact almost all your living space at some point in the future. You can begin to prepare things before the baby is born, but you will also find that you have to be ready to make changes as your child grows.

The Nursery

The big secret about nurseries is that they're not for babies. Instead, their main purpose is to fulfill parents' fantasies. A baby is happy with a bed and somewhere to be changed. Parents are the ones who desire fancy furniture, murals, and accessories. Having a separate room for a baby isn't even strictly necessary. However, having a baby is a big event in your life, and it probably is the fulfillment of your dreams, so making a big to-do out of the nursery is absolutely your right.

When setting up an area for the baby, choose a warm space with natural lighting. Keep the baby's sleeping area away from a window. Child safety experts recommend that you do not use bumper pads, quilts, or heavy blankets in a crib. Hardwood or laminate floors are considered optimal because they don't trap dust and allergens, but many parents prefer carpeting, feeling it is safer should the baby climb out of the crib. If you have an overhead light in the room, install a dimmer switch to make those nighttime diaper changes less startling.

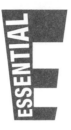

You can find a virtual nursery design tool online to help you design your room at *www.happyhealthypregnancy.com/tools/vr.aspx*. Printing these out can give you a head start on deciding how you want the room arranged.

When planning a baby's room, it is helpful to draw out the room to scale on graph paper. Then you can move around cut-outs of the furniture pieces you'll be using to see where they will best fit.

Baby-Proofing

Like planning a nursery, baby-proofing is something that parents like to do before a baby is born, but it isn't truly necessary, at least not yet. Baby-proofing becomes important once your little one is mobile, but until then most of these steps are not essential. You'll need to add even more safety measures as your child grows and becomes a toddler. If you want to get started with baby-proofing, consider these steps:

- Install outlet covers and hide or shorten electrical cords.
- Cover hard coffee- and end-table corners.
- Install gates on stairs.
- Remove breakable and small items that are within three feet of the floor.
- Adjust your hot-water tank thermostat to below 120 degrees.
- Purchase locks for toilet seat covers.
- Install cabinet door latches.
- Install safety controls on stoves.
- Secure bookcases and tall furniture to the walls.
- Tie up or remove all cords on mini blinds.
- Install bars on windows if you are in a tall building.
- Place child locator decals in the nursery window for firefighters.

Simplifying

Motherhood means juggling lots of things, and the best way to do that is to simplify. There are many things you can do now that will make life easier when the baby arrives:

- Set up a changing area on every floor of your home.
- Start a file to keep warranty information for all your new baby equipment.
- Set up automatic online bill paying and automatic deposit of paychecks if possible.
- Stash basic beauty items (lip gloss, comb, eyeliner, toothbrush, facial wipes) in the room in which you plan on receiving visitors.
- Double every main dish you make from now on and freeze half, so you'll have some meals at the ready.
- Stock up your pantry with nonperishables and create a stockpile of toilet paper, tissues, and other essentials.
- Create a folder of takeout menus and a stash of cash.
- Learn how to use your camera and video recorder before the baby arrives.
- Create a list on which to record baby gifts so you can send thank-you notes.

Making Plans for Help

Asking for help is something a lot of new moms have trouble with, but it makes sense to make plans now for assistance after the baby comes. There are lots of great options available to new moms these days.

Doula

Doulas don't just provide support and assistance during labor and delivery. Postpartum doulas now work for a new mother for weeks and months after birth. These doulas assist with breastfeeding and infant care, as well as episiotomy or C-section incision care. In addition to all of this, they cook, clean, run errands, and more. If your doctor writes a prescription for a postpartum doula, you may be able to get coverage under your health insurance plan.

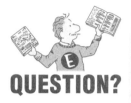

How do I find a postpartum doula?
Contact Doulas of North America (*www.dona.org*; 888-788-3662) for a list of postpartum doulas in your area, or ask your midwife or obstetrician for recommendations.

Baby Nurse

If you would like to hire a nurse who will help with baby care and offer you some relief at night, ask your pediatrician for a recommendation. You can also contact local nanny agencies and ask about specialized baby nurses. Baby nurses will help you with daily baby care and breastfeeding, and they watch the baby during the day or at night so you can sleep or do other things. Note that there are different types of nurses. A registered nurse (RN) will be the most expensive, but if you have a child with special needs this may be necessary. A licensed practical nurse (LPN) does not have the same kind of specialized training as an RN but is well trained to help you with daily care.

Child Care

It's not too soon to begin thinking about child care. Chapter 18 discusses the various options available to you. During your pregnancy you can evaluate day cares for your return to work and get on the waiting list if there is one at the facility you select. Most child-care centers will not take infants younger than six weeks. In addition to making these long-term child-care plans, you should identify friends or relatives who will come over to help so you can sleep or rest in the first months or so that you can have a well-earned parents' night out.

Chapter 11

Protecting Your Family

Preparing for a baby brings many changes that you cannot control. You can't control the physical symptoms of pregnancy, but there are many things you can do to plan ahead for your new family member and the financial impact of becoming a family. Once you become a parent, you suddenly have a family of your own to protect and nurture. Taking the time to do some planning now can help you all feel secure.

Financial Planning

One of the biggest changes a baby brings is right to your bank account. Not only are you facing the costs and expenses of a newborn, but you're also trying to plan for the future—which probably means years of expenses, college, your own retirement, possibly caring for your own parents, and fulfilling your own dreams for yourself.

Financial Goals

To plan for the future, you must first carefully consider your financial goals. Start with your short-term goals. Do you want to buy a house or a new house soon? Do you want to hire a nanny or afford day care? Do you want to take unpaid leave from work? Long-term goals to consider include your career path, private schools, vacation homes, college savings, retirement, and more.

You also need to prioritize your goals. Purchasing a new home may be pressing for you right now, while college savings or retirement may be taking a back seat. It may be helpful to create a list of both your short-term and long-term financial goals. You can place a dollar value on each of the goals and can then use those amounts to help you determine how you will go about reaching them.

Financial Advice

Once you have sorted through your family's financial goals, you need to obtain good advice. It's important to establish a good relationship with a financial advisor whom you can rely upon and trust. If you don't have a financial planner, you can ask for a referral from a family member or friend, or you can call your local financial planners' association.

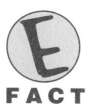

FACT

There are several types of financial planner designations. Certified financial planners, chartered financial planners, personal financial specialists, and registered financial consultants all take different licensing exams. Some planners charge a fee, while others take only commission.

Your financial planner can help you look at your financial goals realistically and help you develop an overall financial plan that will allow you to meet them. This may include taking a look at your savings strategy, your retirement needs, college costs, investment vehicles, and spending habits. Another important consideration your planner will discuss is the type of risk you want to assume in an investment. If you are planning for a retirement that is thirty years away, you may be comfortable with higher-risk investments that may have a greater payoff over a long period of time. If on the other hand you are planning for the short term, you may feel more comfortable with low-risk investments.

Your Child's Financial Future

Another important financial consideration is whether you want to start to build a financial base for your child. Many parents open bank accounts for their child. If you're interested in doing so, there are two types to consider. A Uniform Gift to Minors Act (UGMA) account is in the child's name with the parent as custodian. The parent has complete control of the account until the child reaches 18 or 21 (depending on your state's laws). Another option is a Uniform Transfers to Minors Act (UTMA) account, which allows a parent to retain control of the account until the child completes college. Deposits of up to $750 per year are tax-free until the child is age 14. If people write checks to the baby, you can sign them and deposit them in the account yourself. Your child will need to have a social security number before you can open a bank account or other investment vehicle in his or her name.

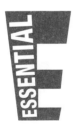

If you invest 70 cents per day from the day your baby is born, he or she will be a millionaire by age 65. Starting to create savings for your child early on can offer him financial security later in life.

You may also wish to open an investment or individual retirement account (IRA) for your child now. If your child's investment earns more than $1,600 a year, the income will be taxed at the same rate as your own income.

Health Insurance and Medical Savings Accounts

Health insurance is one of the most important financial tools available to your family because it protects you from catastrophic medical expenses. Unfortunately, the cost of health care and health insurance continues to rise, making it a very large expense. This can be true even if you are only contributing to the cost and your employer or partner's employer is paying for a majority of the premium. Now that you will have a child, it makes sense to go with a family plan, rather than you and your partner each carrying a separate policy. All of you can be covered under the family plan. If your or your partner's employer pays the full cost of insurance, but you choose the other person's plan to use as a family plan, you may wish to continue holding the individual policy.

Make sure you have a complete understanding of your health insurance plan, and when it is time to choose a plan, weigh the options carefully. Note that you can add your child onto the policy at the date of birth and do not need to wait for an enrollment period. Now that you are going to be a parent, things such as coverage for well visits, vaccinations, and sick visit co-pays will be important. Checking on coverage for nontraditional providers is also important if you or your partner see a chiropractor or if you plan to use a doula for your birth. Some prescription plans allow you to obtain substantial deductions on prescriptions through a mail-order program, so you may also want to weigh that factor when you are evaluating policies.

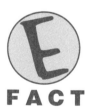

FACT

In 2004, 8.3 million U.S. children did not have health insurance—11.2 percent of all kids. Fortunately, many states now have health insurance programs that are provided at no cost or on a sliding scale for children and parents. Contact your state department of social services for information or visit *www.insurekidsnow.gov*.

Pay attention to your health-care plan's rules for out-of-network providers. Using an in-network provider can be a substantial savings. In addition, requirements for referrals are important. If you or your child needs a referral to see a specialist and you do not obtain it before the appointment, you may not be able to have it backdated and will be responsible for the full cost of the visit. Note that most plans usually do not require a referral to see an OB/GYN or a midwife, nor does your child need one for a pediatrician if you select one as her primary-care provider.

Health Savings Accounts

A health savings account, or HSA, is designed to be used only in conjunction with health care. If you have a high-deductible health plan (one that meets requirements for minimum family and individual deductibles), you qualify to set up and use one of these accounts. As of this writing, the law allows you to contribute up to $2,600 pre-tax dollars per year as an individual or $5,150 as a family. The funds in the account must be used to pay for health expenses. Because you deposit the money before taxes, it is never taxed, meaning you get a substantial savings when you use this money. Your financial advisor can set up an HSA for you, and you can decide how to invest the money so that it will grow.

If you do not use the entire balance of the account in a year, the money remains in the account and can be used in the future. If you withdraw money from the account and use it for a nonmedical expense, you have to pay tax on it, as well as a 10 percent penalty. When using an HSA, it is essential that you keep good records. You need to be able to provide a receipt for every withdrawal you make from the account to prove it was used for a medical expense.

Flexible Spending Account

A flexible spending account (FSA) is set up by your employer. You deposit pre-tax dollars in the account via payroll deduction—up to $5,000 per year, per family. The funds in the account can be used to pay for medical expenses, including over-the-counter medications and fertility treatments. Unlike an HSA, an FSA is a use-it-or-lose-it option. If you do not use the money in your FSA by the end of the year (there is an extension of two months and fifteen days after the end of the calendar year), you forfeit the entire unspent amount. Because of this, you need to carefully plan your foreseeable medical expenses and contribute up to that amount.

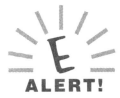

ALERT!

Studies show that workers on average forfeit $100 per year by leaving unused funds in a flexible spending account. If you approach the end of the year and have money left, get your teeth cleaned or an eye exam, stock up on over-the-counter medications, or encourage your partner to go in for a checkup.

Pregnancy and new parenthood are a good time to make use of an FSA because you will have a lot of planned health care expenses, including prenatal checkups, ultrasounds, prenatal vitamins, childbirth classes, hospital co-pays, well-baby visits, and more. Pay attention to when in the calendar year your due date falls. Depending on when you have your baby, you may need to spread your FSA contributions over two calendar years to maximize it.

FSAs can also be used to pay for child-care costs, including day-care centers, nannies, and other professional child-care workers who have tax ID numbers.

Wills

A will is a very important document that will not only direct how your belongings will be divided should you die but will also determine guardianship for your child. According to U.S. probate court statistics, most people—70 percent—die without a will. Having one prepared is neither expensive nor difficult.

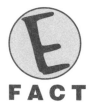

FACT

To find an attorney who specializes in wills and estates, get a referral from your local bar association or contact the American Academy of Estate Planning Attorneys (online at *www.aaepa.com*; 800-846-1555).

Requirements for wills are different in every state, so it is important to have an attorney draw one up for you. You can meet with an attorney during your pregnancy and have a will drawn up, but you should consult with your attorney about whether you can sign it before the birth of your child.

When selecting a guardian for your child, choose someone who would raise your child in a way most compatible with your own style and who is able to take on the responsibility. For many people, this is a close relative or friend who will have an ongoing relationship with the child throughout his or her life. It's a good idea to choose an alternate guardian in case your first choice is not available or cannot take on the responsibility. Your selection of a guardian will most likely be upheld by the court should appointing a guardian ever be necessary; however, the judge has discretion to make a choice that seems best.

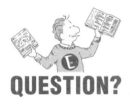

QUESTION?

Why do I need a will if state laws will divide my property without one?

If you die without a will (called dying intestate), your belongings are divided according to a formula your state uses (dividing things among spouse and children primarily), not according to your own particular wishes. And if you die without a will, you can't formally make your wishes about guardianship known to the court.

Health-Care Directives

A health-care directive is a legal document that states what kind of treatment you would choose for yourself in a situation in which you are unable to communicate, such as unconscious, in a coma, or under anesthesia.

This can include directions about life-sustaining treatment, pain management, food and hydration, and more. Additionally, the document may appoint someone who can make health-care decisions for you if you are not able.

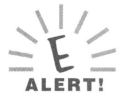

A health-care directive is only useful if your spouse or family member is able to find it and produce it when needed. Don't keep this document in a bank safe-deposit box; instead, store it at home or use the online U.S. Living Will Registry (*www.uslivingwillregistry.com*).

There are a variety of different health-care directives, and the requirements are different in every state. You should see an attorney to have one drawn up that will meet your state requirements. During pregnancy is a good time to have a health-care directive drawn up so that you can feel fully prepared should you face a C-section or other medical intervention.

Life Insurance

Life insurance is another long-term plan that many people wish to make when they become parents. When you buy life insurance, you pay a yearly premium. In exchange, upon your death, the company pays the face amount of your policy to your beneficiary. You can choose your spouse or child as a beneficiary, as well as other relatives.

There are many types of life insurance, including some that also function as investments. Some experts believe it makes more sense to invest money in secure investments rather than to buy life insurance. On the other hand, many people simply don't feel certain that their loved ones will be secure without life insurance; talk with your own financial advisor about what might be best for you. Many people choose a mix of life insurance and other investments.

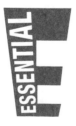

When considering life insurance, be sure to get information on the face value as well as the cash value of the policy—two different things. Ask to see a net payment index that will clearly show the costs of the policy, as well as the surrender cost index.

It's not usually advisable for a woman to buy life insurance during pregnancy. (She's considered to be at higher risk of health problems, and thus the cost is higher.) But your partner can, and you can purchase insurance shortly after the birth if you have not purchased any prior to becoming pregnant.

College Savings

Saving for college is one of the biggest things parents worry about, but when you're pregnant or caring for a newborn, the need can seem far-off. Although you have eighteen years to find the money for college, starting to plan now can give you a big head start on the huge costs involved.

There are many ways to save for college. Before your baby is born, it probably makes sense to start a generalized savings plan, where you place money into a money market or other interest-bearing account. You can use these funds for a variety of things, such as baby equipment, a down payment on a new home, a minivan, and so on, as well as the beginning of a college nest egg.

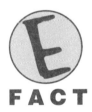

FACT

At the present time, on average, it costs $5,500 per year for a four-year public college and $21,000 per year for a four-year private college education, not including room and board. College costs are rising at a rate of about 8 percent per year.

Once your baby is born, you may wish to begin a formal college savings plan. There are two types of college savings plans, but it is important to remember that you can save money for college without placing it in one of these kinds of accounts. It is important to talk to your financial planner about the options available to you and your family.

529 Plans

A 529, or Qualified Tuition Plan, is a savings plan with tax advantages to help students save money for college costs. Each state sponsors its own

529 plan, and each is different, so you will need to do research and some comparison-shopping before you decide on one.

There are two types of 529 plans. One is prepaid. Under this type of plan, you pay your child's tuition at current prices. This can be a good deal, considering that college costs are always rising. However, this type of plan only guarantees tuition at an in-state public college. If your child goes out of state or attends a private college, you'll be able to apply the cash value to tuition, but it won't be fully paid. The other type of 529 is a savings plan, in which you add funds to the account and it slowly grows over the years. When your child goes to college, these funds can then be used for expenses.

Funds placed in a 529 plan are not taxed, and interest is tax exempt. Most accounts can be opened with a very small initial investment, as little as $25. The money in the account can be used to pay for tuition, room and board, books, and other college costs. If the funds are used for other purposes, there is a 10 percent penalty. You can create an automatic monthly transfer to the account from your bank account if you want it automated, or you can make deposits whenever you wish. The caps on the contribution levels are quite high; research each individual plan to find out its limits. Another way to make contributions, at no cost to yourself, is to sign up for a plan like Upromise (*www.upromise.com*). You register your credit cards and grocery cards with the plan. and when you purchase qualifying products, you earn money that is transferred to your 529 plan. Grandparents can also sign up to have their credits go to your child's account.

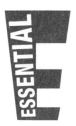

Even if you don't have immediate plans to contribute to a college savings account, it makes sense to open one as soon as your baby is born. Relatives and friends can then contribute to the plan as baby gifts.

Some parents worry they will create a college savings account and their child will choose not to go to college. In that case, funds from a 529 plan can be transferred to another family member. Additionally, if your child does not go to college, you can simply refund the money in the account to yourself, less the penalty.

When choosing a 529 plan, it is important to shop around. Just because you live in New York, for example, you do not need to sign up with the New York plan. Most plans do not require that you use the money at a school within that state, so your child will not be restricted to a college in any particular state.

Coverdell Education Savings

Coverdell Education Savings Accounts (also called Coverdell ESAs) were previously called education IRAs. This type of plan allows the parent to control where and how the money is invested. This is different from a 529 plan, where you choose a plan and the plan administrators manage your investment. You can contribute up to $2,000 per year, per child. This limit applies no matter how many accounts your child has. For example, if you open one and a grandparent each open one, the total added to both accounts cannot exceed $2,000 in one year.

The money placed in the account is not taxed as long you meet certain income requirements (currently, joint income must be under $190,000 and individual income must be under $95,000). The funds in a Coverdell ESA are not taxed if they total less than the child's total education costs (including elementary and secondary schools, as well as colleges and universities).

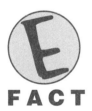

FACT

Paying for college may seem like a huge burden, but most college students today don't rely on their parents to pay their way. 63 percent of college students in 2004 received some kind of financial aid. A college education definitely pays off, with college graduates earning an average of $46,000 per year, compared to the average of $27,000 per year for high school graduates.

Coverdell funds can be used for tuition, books, and school fees. Funds used for other purposes are taxed and subjected to a 10 percent penalty. You cannot contribute to the account after the child reaches age 18, and the money in the account must be used before the child turns 30. Money remaining in the account after this point becomes property of the child and cannot be refunded to the parent. You can contribute to both a Coverdell ESA and a 529 plan simultaneously.

Cord Blood Preservation

Cord blood is blood from the umbilical cord, which contains stem cells. Cord blood preservation is something many parents are interested in and that they see as a way to obtain peace of mind about their child's future health.

The Importance of Cord Blood

Stem cells are considered important because they can be used in the treatment of at least forty-five diseases (according to the American Pregnancy Association). Many families choose to preserve their child's cord blood should it ever be needed to treat a disease developed by the child. Cord blood is more compatible than blood from family members or unrelated donors. It can be used not only for the child but also for other family members. There is a 25 percent chance of a match for a sibling.

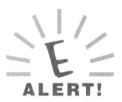

Despite the popularity of cord blood preservation, the American Academy of Pediatrics (AAP) recommends that parents bank their child's blood only if there is a family member with a current or potential need for a stem cell transplant. In other cases, the AAP calls cord blood storage "unwise."

Companies that store cord blood advocate the process because the umbilical cord stem cells are genetically identical to the baby from whose placenta they were derived, and stem cells in general have a lower risk of rejection should a stem cell transplant be needed. The problem with cord blood has to do with genetics. Most diseases that would benefit from stem cell transplantation have a genetic basis. In those cases, the stem cells from the cord blood would harbor the same genetic disease and would not be useful.

Additionally, the chances of a child needing a stem cell transplant is very small, about one in 1,400. On the other hand, umbilical cord stem cells derived from public banks can and have been used in many instances and show great promise. Because of all of this, many authorities feel that there is not a compelling case for private banking of umbilical cord blood. At the same time, the case for donating of umbilical cord stem cells to public banks is excellent.

Harvesting Cord Blood

Cord blood is harvested from the umbilical cord when the cord is cut after birth. A needle is used to drain the cord blood, and there is no pain involved for mother or baby. The container holding the blood is then transported to a special storage facility. Often the blood is tested upon arrival, and a report is sent to the parents.

Cord Blood Contracts

If you decide that you want your baby's cord blood harvested and preserved, you need to make arrangements while you are pregnant, well before the birth. You should research the companies that offer this service, select one, sign a contract, and make financial arrangements. The average cost of a cord blood contract is $1,500 up front plus a storage fee of $100 per month. You need to obtain the cord blood collection kit and make sure it comes with you to the hospital or birth center. The hospital staff will handle the collection, and the cord blood company arranges for transport of the specimen.

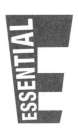

If you're interested in cord blood donation, contact the National Cord Blood Donation Program (*www.nationalcordbloodprogram.com*). Just as there is a national supply of blood, contributing to the program will help build a national supply of cord blood. It costs you nothing while giving you the knowledge that you are helping build a supply that anyone can use.

If you decide to bank your baby's blood, make sure that you get a clear explanation of all fees and that all services are described in full. Ask about mechanisms that are in place to preserve the blood in case of power failure, natural disaster, or closure of the facility. Choose a facility that is registered with the U.S. Food and Drug Administration and fully accredited by the American Association of Tissue Banks. Find out how you can withdraw blood and what documentation is needed to make that request.

Chapter 12

Feeling Good Throughout Your Pregnancy

Pregnancy is an ever-changing condition. One minute you're sick, the next you're not. One minute you're excited, the next you're terrified. Staying focused and remaining positive will help you feel better mentally and physically throughout your pregnancy.

Managing Stress

During your pregnancy, you're dealing with a lot of changes, as well as the thought of many more changes to come in the future. You are probably thrilled to experience these changes. At the same time, it can be very stressful to manage all of these new things and cope with the physical limitations you may be encountering.

Several studies have shown that very high levels of stress can contribute to preterm birth and low birth weights in babies. Note that we're not talking about everyday momentary stress, such as getting a little upset in traffic or feeling bad because you flubbed a presentation. This is ongoing high-level stress, the kind that is unhealthy for anyone. Ongoing stress during pregnancy can cause fatigue, problems sleeping, lack of appetite, overeating, headaches, and backaches. While some stress is unavoidable, controlling the stress levels in your life can help you feel better during pregnancy.

Physical Stresses

Pregnancy is all about your changing body. It can be very frustrating to suddenly feel as though your entire life is ruled by your physical condition. You do have to listen to your body during pregnancy, but you don't have to let it stop you from doing the things that are important to you. Pregnancy stress and mood swings are often caused in part by blood sugar changes, hormonal fluctuations, and even water retention. Mood swings tend to even out midway through pregnancy, but many women experience them until the baby is born.

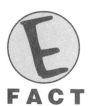

FACT

According to the American Society for Reproductive Medicine, a woman under age 30 has a 20 percent chance of pregnancy each month. At age 40, a woman has only a 5 percent chance of pregnancy each month.

Learning to manage the physical demands of pregnancy means changing your expectations. You can still do almost all of the things you enjoy, but you may need to modify them. For example, if you've always loved hiking, you can still do it, but you may need to take more frequent breaks, go shorter distances, or choose less-challenging paths. Make compromises with yourself and your pregnancy that you can do the physical things you want to do in a way that keeps your body comfortable and healthy.

Surprise Stressors

Pregnancy can make your emotions unpredictable and unstable at times. Things that have never bothered you can suddenly become unbearable. For reasons you can't explain, or even understand yourself, a small annoyance can erupt into what feels like a crisis. While these unexpected upsets can definitely keep you on your toes, they can also make you feel like a giant heap of uncontrolled hormones.

Accept that sometimes you will unexpectedly find yourself crying or angry about things that previously might not have made a hill of beans of difference to you. Part of the difficulty in these situations is that you feel frustrated at yourself for reacting in a way that might seem uncharacteristic. It can be difficult to relinquish control of your emotions to your pregnancy, but struggling against it can actually create more internal stress. You're not losing your mind or becoming out of control if you find that your emotions overwhelm you during pregnancy; you're simply reacting to the signals your body is sending out.

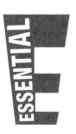

If you and your partner do not share a last name, you may be wondering what name your baby can have. You can choose either name, a combination, or a completely different last name for your baby. You do so simply by entering this on the birth certificate application.

Stress Relief Techniques

One of the keys to coping with stress is to pinpoint what exactly is bothering you. Many times there may be nothing specific because your hormones are simply making you weepy, but sometimes there are specific triggers that you can identify and then work on. Whether you are worried about a project at work, upset because the nursery hasn't been painted, feeling neglected by your partner, or are overtired, you can best cope with the stress if you're able to first isolate its cause. Once you have done that, work to reduce, resolve, or eliminate the problem. Of course, many problems can't be made to go away, and so there are some things you have to learn to cope with.

To help relieve and reduce your stress during pregnancy, do the following:

- Eat healthy meals and snacks regularly, and drink enough water.
- Exercise regularly, if your health-care provider approves.
- Get enough sleep, and rest when you need to.
- Avoid caffeine and alcohol, which are not considered acceptable during pregnancy and can add to your stress.
- Try soothing techniques, such as yoga, massage, meditation, baths, or other activities that bring you joy and pleasure. Breathing exercises or medication can also be very relaxing.
- Talk to friends and family about the things that are bothering you. Bottling stress up inside of you only makes it worse.

Remember that all pregnancy-related stresses are temporary. Pregnancy doesn't last forever, and your life is in an intense period of change. What seems unbearable today may become a mere blip on your radar tomorrow. Remind yourself that you will get through this, and you will work through anything that is troubling or bothering you.

Dealing with Worries and Fears

At some point, just about every pregnant woman worries about whether her baby will be okay, and she feels nervous about birth. These are normal reactions to pregnancy. While they can make you feel unsettled, they are not something you should dwell on.

The whole point of your pregnancy is to have a healthy baby, and most women are well aware that there are many things that can go wrong. However, the odds are that you will have a healthy baby. Your health-care provider can help ease your fears. It's his job to help make sure that your baby grows well and comes into the world healthy. Some health-care providers tell their patients to let them worry about the unlikely possibilities and ask the patient to keep her mind focused on enjoying pregnancy.

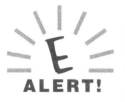

Some studies have shown that women with extremely stressful jobs are at a higher risk for preeclampsia, a dangerous high blood pressure condition in pregnancy. If you have a job that is very high pressure, talk to your health-care provider about what you can do to ensure a healthy pregnancy.

If you've never given birth before, labor and delivery is a new thing for you. New experiences are always a little frightening simply because you can't completely know what to expect in advance. If you are fearful or nervous about birth, the best thing you can do is take a childbirth preparation class. The class will provide you with a lot of information and help you talk through your fears. You will also learn techniques that will put you in control during labor and delivery and help you manage your fears at that time.

Talking to other moms may help with your fears, or it may make them worse. Don't talk to people who are intent on sharing their horror stories with you. Remember that each woman is different. Your experience will be your own, not a re-enactment of someone else's. Talking to your health-care provider can also ease your worries. Let her know what aspect of birth you are most worried about, and she can talk you through it and help you understand that she will be there to help you get through it.

Sex and Intimacy

It's ironic that intercourse is what begins a pregnancy and then becomes something many women aren't very interested in. There are lots of ways to stay connected to your partner during pregnancy, and intercourse is only one of them.

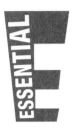

Talk to your health-care provider about any restrictions on your sex life. If you experience vaginal bleeding, leak amniotic fluid, have an incompetent cervix, are having preterm labor, have a history of miscarriages, or are having problems with your pregnancy, intercourse is not recommended.

Sexual intimacy and sex are safe throughout pregnancy, all the way to end. It cannot hurt the baby, who is not aware of what you are doing. Having orgasms does not cause you to go into labor or have a miscarriage. Orgasms can sometimes cause uterine contractions, though. In an otherwise-normal pregnancy, this poses no risk. However, if your pregnancy is at high risk for premature labor or delivery, it is not clear if orgasms that cause contractions may pose a risk; you should speak with your health-care provider.

However, just because sex is safe doesn't mean it's at the top of the list for some women. In early pregnancy, nausea and fatigue can play a big part in reducing a woman's interest in sex. During the second trimester, interest in sex often returns, sometimes very strongly. During the third trimester, backache, fatigue, and the size of the uterus can make sex again become complicated. Many moms will tell you that sex can work to relieve some of your symptoms and can be a great way to relax during pregnancy.

Some women feel nervous about sexual intercourse during the first trimester because they worry it may cause miscarriage. This may especially be true for women who have a problem with repetitive miscarriages or who have had fertility problems. Although there is no evidence that intercourse causes miscarriage, many women still are apprehensive. If this is something you are worried about, it's perfectly fine to hold off on intercourse until you have an ultrasound or until the first trimester is over.

Oral sex is safe during pregnancy, as long as your partner does not blow air into your vagina. The air may enter the large blood vessels that supply the vagina and cervix and travel to the heart; this is called an air embolism, and can be fatal. Anal intercourse during pregnancy is not dangerous, but due to engorgement of the hemorrhoidal veins or hemorrhoids during pregnancy, it may be uncomfortable or may cause bleeding.

Sex toys are something many women wonder about and on which there is no clear consensus. If sex toys are not cleaned meticulously, they can cause infection. If they are inserted too deeply or too forcefully, they can cause injury. If you would like to use sex toys during pregnancy, it's a good idea to talk with your health-care provider first. Don't be embarrassed to discuss this. Any health-care provider will be happy to talk about this and would much prefer to have a frank, unembarrassed conversation than have a patient sustain an injury.

No sexual activity (penile penetration, sex toy, or oral sex) should ever involve going from the anal orifice to the vagina since this can introduce infection. Some women find that pregnancy greatly increases their sex drive. If you experience this, it is completely normal. The hormonal fluctuations of pregnancy play a part in how interested you are in sex.

Because there is increased blood supply to vaginal and cervical tissues during pregnancy, mild vaginal bleeding or spotting may occur after intercourse, especially if the penis bumps against the cervix during sex. If this occurs after sex, don't panic; it does not hurt the baby. You should, however, always contact your health-care provider immediately if any bleeding occurs during pregnancy regardless of the circumstances.

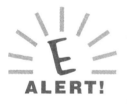
ALERT!

If your partner has oral or genital herpes, you need to talk to your health-care provider about avoiding transmission since contracting herpes during pregnancy can be very dangerous to the baby. Remember that herpes can be transmitted even if your partner is not experiencing symptoms.

Nipple stimulation can definitely cause contractions and even induce labor in the third trimester. The effect can be as powerful as the drug oxcytocin which is used to induce labor. Because of this, excessive nipple stimulation should be avoided during pregnancy. This is especially important in pregnancies already at risk for premature delivery.

If you find you're not interested in intercourse, you and your partner can satisfy each other in other ways. It's important to remember that you can find ways to feel close to your partner that do not involve intercourse or sexual behavior. Just spending time together, holding hands, having him rub your back, or doing things together to prepare for the baby can give you a sense of closeness and connectedness.

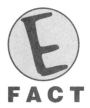

FACT

In a survey done by Babycenter.com, 40 percent of women surveyed said that pregnancy drastically reduced the amount of sex they were having. For tips and good advice, read *Hot Mamas: The Ultimate Guide to Staying Sexy Throughout Your Pregnancy and the Months Beyond*, by Lou Paget.

Some women worry that their partner will no longer find them to be attractive as their body changes throughout pregnancy. Usually this is an unfounded worry. A loving and caring partner loves you for who you are and is thrilled to watch as the child develops. Many men find pregnant women beautiful and attractive at every stage. If this is something you're worried about, talk about it with your partner. Find out how he is feeling, and share your own concerns or worries. It is likely you will be able to find a way to keep both of you satisfied and happy throughout your pregnancy.

Another concern of many women is that giving birth will permanently change their vagina so that sex will never be the same again. The vagina is able to stretch and retract. While having a baby does change your body, it does not mean you'll never enjoy sex again or that your partner will not find as much pleasure in you after you have a baby. Wait until after your postpartum checkup before having sex.

Coping with Pregnancy Problems

Hopefully, your pregnancy will go smoothly, but even if you encounter some problems, you can still get through them and have a healthy baby. A wide variety of problems or complications can arise in a pregnancy. Your health-care provider can manage and control most of these.

It's important to remember that most pregnancy problems are minor. Puffy ankles might not be fun, but most of the time they aren't extremely serious. Because you're getting good medical care, your health-care provider will be able to spot problems and take steps to reduce any risks.

Blame

It's not uncommon for women to blame themselves for things that go wrong during pregnancy. "I must have done something to cause this," or "There are things I could have done that would have prevented this from happening" are common thoughts. What you must realize, though, is there is most likely nothing you did or didn't do that brought about whatever problem you are experiencing. Remind yourself of all the things you've done to stay healthy—seen a health-care provider, eaten healthy foods, and avoided drugs, tobacco, and alcohol.

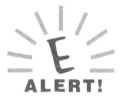
ALERT!

After the fourth month of pregnancy, a woman should not lie flat on her back because the weight of the uterus places pressure on blood vessels. Because of this, the missionary position is not recommended for sex after the fourth month of pregnancy.

Blaming yourself is not helpful. It doesn't really matter what exactly caused your complication to arise since you can't change what has happened. What you can do, however, is move forward with your health-care provider to resolve the complication and ensure that you will have an uneventful end to your pregnancy.

Bed Rest

According to the *Online Journal of Health Ethics*, 20 percent of women are placed on bed rest for at least one week of their pregnancy. Being put on bed rest is difficult and worrisome. The first thing you need to do is find out exactly what activities are permitted and which are not. There are many different degrees of bed rest, and it is important to get details about what is safe for you to do. Ask your health-care provider about these possibilities:

- Working from home
- Lifting children
- Performing daily household activities
- Climbing stairs
- Walking around and mobility in general
- Showering and bathing
- Sitting versus lying down
- Driving a car
- Having sex and experiencing orgasm
- Stretching and light exercise
- Watching for warning signs

If you are restricted and told to stay home and put your feet up, or stay in bed, there are some things you can do to make it more bearable. Set yourself up in a room that provides everything you need within arm's reach. A bed and a recliner may be allowed. You will probably want access to a TV, DVD player, CD player, computer, and telephone. Stay in touch with friends and family by encouraging them to visit and by talking on the phone. This is a good time to read books you've had on your nightstand for a while or to take up a hobby such as knitting, scrapbooking, or learning to play chess. Look at this time as a time of rest and rejuvenation and a chance to focus on your pregnancy and your baby.

Managing Health Problems

If you experience a complication in your pregnancy, the most important thing to do is to follow your health-care provider's instructions. It's very easy to go online and do research yourself. While educating yourself is a great idea, self-diagnosis and treatment are not. If you come across things online that concern you, ask your health-care provider about them before doing anything.

Remember that health-care concerns are a physical situation but also a mental and emotional one. It takes time and mental and emotional effort to cope with a complication. You cannot expect yourself to not feel any effects, no matter how minor a complication you are experiencing. You need to give yourself time and space to think things through, ask questions, and care for yourself.

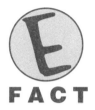

FACT

The risk for preeclampsia is higher for women having their first baby at an older age. For this reason, your health-care provider will always check your blood pressure and test your ankles for swelling. Rapid weight gain (more than two to three pounds in a week) may also be a warning sign of preeclampsia.

Finding Support

The good news about pregnancy is that lots and lots of women are going through it or have gone through it. You are by no means alone. Talking with other moms or pregnant women can help you feel less anxious and can offer important connections. The nurses, midwives, or physicians at your health-care provider can also offer support and information.

There are lots of ways to get in touch with other pregnant women, if you are interested. Joining a prenatal exercise or yoga class can help you get to know other pregnant women in your area. When you take your childbirth education class, you will meet other women who have due dates close to yours. Since you are all roughly at the same stage of pregnancy, you can go through it all together and learn from and support each other.

Many women find support online. There are myriad bulletin boards and listservs for pregnant moms. You can join due-date clubs, where all the women on a board or list are due in the same month. Many of these lists stay together for years, as the women support each other through different stages of motherhood. There are also many boards and lists for particular interests—over 35, plus-size, pregnant again after a loss, gestational diabetes, and so on.

Don't forget to rely on your partner, family, and friends for support. Although they may not be going through a pregnancy, they love you and are there to listen and help you. Your health-care provider's staff is not only very educated about pregnancy but also very interested in helping women through all aspects of it. There is sure to be someone there who can help you with almost any problem.

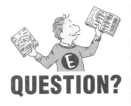

QUESTION?

How do I find online pregnancy support groups?
One good place to start is *www.babycenter.com/bbs*, where you can explore a wide variety of bulletin boards. Almost all pregnancy and parenting Web sites have similar boards. If you are interested in a listserv, where you communicate by e-mail, go to *www.yahoogroups.com* and search for pregnancy.

Working While Pregnant

Because each job, and each woman, is different, there are no hard-and-fast rules about working during pregnancy. Whatever is right for you, in your situation, is the right answer. There will be times throughout your pregnancy when working will be a challenge, but working while pregnant does not have to be difficult.

Pregnancy Discrimination

One of the most important things to know is that your employer cannot tell you to stop working or change your job responsibilities because you are pregnant. Employers cannot refuse to hire a woman, fire her, or refuse to promote her simply because she is pregnant. The Pregnancy Discrimination Act is a federal law that protects a woman's right to work while pregnant and prohibits these discriminatory practices.

Although there is a law prohibiting discrimination against pregnant women, it's simply a well-known fact that many employers view pregnancy as the first step onto the mommy track. You can avoid this by making clear your commitment to your job and making plans that show you will continue to be an important employee after you return from maternity leave.

Staying Comfortable While Working

As you may already know, pregnancy is not always the most comfortable of conditions. You may tire easily, your feet may ache, your back may hurt, you may get hungry or nauseous, you may feel hot, and so on. These things are hard enough to manage at home, but when you're working they can be even more troublesome.

Don't be afraid to ask for accommodations at your place of employment. If you need to sit more, do so. If traveling has become difficult for you, cut back. If your work area is too hot, ask for a change or more ventilation. Pregnancy does not have to change how well you do your job, but it may have to change how you physically perform your job functions. If you are experiencing problems with nausea at certain times of the day, build your schedule around that. If you find you have no energy at a certain time of the day, try to work around that. Remind yourself that any changes you make are temporary. If your job requires you to work around dangerous chemicals or in dangerous conditions, you are within your rights to ask for a change in job responsibilities during your pregnancy.

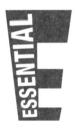

If you sit at a desk at work, make sure you are using a chair that has good lumbar support during your pregnancy. You may also wish to bring in a small footstool, or even a box, to put under your desk so that you can put your feet up. Getting up and stretching frequently will also help relieve discomfort.

Wear comfortable clothes and shoes that are professional but that also feel good and do not cause you discomfort. Avoid clothes that are too hot or too tight. Shoes that are too tight or too high are likely to cause you problems as well. Bring snacks to work with you, and make sure you eat and drink frequently, even if this is something you never used to make time for before pregnancy. Build rests into your day so that you have a few moments to recharge.

Time off Work During Pregnancy

There may be times in your pregnancy when you simply do not feel well or are directed to stay off your feet or in bed. You can use your sick and vacation leave for these times, but you also can take unpaid time off under the Family and Medical Leave Act (FMLA). The law allows women to take time off for their own health care problems (as well as time off to care for a newborn, as described in Chapter 10). There are up to twelve weeks per twelve-month period available to you under this law. However if you use the full twelve weeks during pregnancy, you don't get another twelve weeks when the baby comes. You may also be able to take time off under a state family and medical leave law, so consult your human resources department.

Talk to your human resources department and get information about pregnancy disability pay. You may be eligible for this if your physician says it is medically necessary for you to stop working during pregnancy.

Making Time for Medical Appointments

All the medical appointments necessary during pregnancy—prenatal checkups, lab work, ultrasounds, and other tests—can be time-consuming and difficult to work into an already-busy schedule. If your schedule is extremely tight, you may want to work with a health-care provider who makes appointments early in the morning (before 9 A.M.) or on Saturdays. Many labs are open for blood draws on Saturdays and very early in the morning, and many take appointments.

Some procedures almost always have to be scheduled during normal business hours, such as ultrasounds and other tests. You may want to try to schedule these appointments into your lunch hour. Your employer may be flexible and allow you to work later to make up for time out of the workplace during the day if you need to miss work to make an appointment. If none of these options works for you, you may have no choice but to use sick or personal time for these appointments. If so, call before you leave for the appointment to make sure the office or provider is running on time so you don't waste time in a waiting room.

Chapter 13

Loving Your Pregnant Self

With the busyness and exhaustion of pregnancy, it is sometimes easy to lose sight of the one person who needs you the most—yourself. You should embrace your changing body and changing psyche throughout pregnancy. This is a life-changing experience, and one that you should enjoy, rather than simply tolerate, counting the days until it is over.

Dealing with Body Changes

In a society that emphasizes appearance, and worships thinness, it can be difficult to watch helplessly as not only your abdomen expands but as you also see changes to almost every other part of your body. Learning to accept and love a larger body can be a challenge for many women.

Pregnancy can be difficult to adjust to for women who have struggled with body image all their lives, but it can be equally difficult for women who have never had conflicting feelings about their body. Whether you've always been thin, have always been overweight, or have yo-yoed, it can be difficult to embrace your new shape. Perhaps the thing that is most frustrating is that suddenly your body is out of your control. People are used to controlling and shaping their bodies through exercise and diet, but in pregnancy, you can't prevent change.

Some women are really displeased with the changes in their body and think themselves to be fat, misshapen, or unattractive. Other women thoroughly enjoy pregnancy, reveling in their new shape and enjoying the fact that for once in their lives they do not have to struggle to retain their figure.

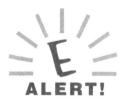

ALERT!

If you have an eating disorder, it is essential that you tell your health-care provider. Failing to eat enough, or eating and purging, can deprive your baby of essential nutrients, and you could face miscarriage, pre-term labor, birth defects, or a low birth weight baby. If you are an over-eater, it is also important that you work with your health-care provider to limit your weight gain.

If you are feeling uncomfortable with your burgeoning body, or the prospect of pregnancy changes yet to come, there are things you can do to continue to feel good about yourself and your physical changes. First, take positive steps for your health. Doing things that are good for your body, such as exercising and eating healthy foods, will make you feel good physically and will give you a mental and emotional boost.

Take the time to remember that your body is performing a miracle. Appreciate the miracle, even if you aren't so pleased with the outward consequences. Remember that every pound you gain is another important benefit to your baby and that as your body changes, so does your baby. Your baby loves you and your body exactly the way it is.

Try to focus on the pregnant glow you're giving off, and accentuate the parts of your body that you appreciate. Many women are excited to see their breasts get larger, for example. Touching your own body will help you feel more comfortable with it, and the tactile connection will bring together your body and your mind. Try to be accepting and appreciative of the changes you experience, and remember there are many women who cannot ever experience this. Pregnancy is giving the gift of your body to another human being. Once the pregnancy is over, you can start to regain your body—the gift is not permanent.

Accepting That You Must Do Less

For many women who have lives that are happily full with careers, relationships, friends, activities, and interests, it can sometimes be difficult to let pregnancy step in and slow them down. It's easy to say to yourself that pregnancy won't change anything and while having a baby may require some minor adjustments, everything in life can go on as it did before. However, the truth is that pregnancy does require changes, and being a mother is more life-altering than you think it will be.

Just because you are pregnant you don't need to quit your job, cancel your gym membership, and relegate yourself to the recliner all day. It's important to stay active, do the things you love, and follow your interests during pregnancy. However, the simple fact is that there will be days when you're tired, sick, puffy, cranky, weepy, or just huge. And on these days, you will find that your previous schedule just doesn't cut it.

If you try and push yourself, refusing to yield to the needs of your changing body, you will probably find yourself extremely tired and overwhelmed. Your body has taken on a gigantic project of its own, and it needs some of your focus and energy to complete it. Thinking that pregnancy doesn't have to have an impact on your life at all is not realistic.

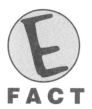

A study done in Poland found that heavy physical labor at work during pregnancy was linked to low birth-weight babies, whereas simply expending a lot of energy at work was not as clear a risk factor for low birth weight. The study showed that pregnant women need to be careful when it comes to heavy work, but there is no danger in using a lot of energy during pregnancy.

You can continue to do everything you want to do, but in moderation. Or you may find there are some things you want to cut out of your life to make more room for other things that are more important to you. For example, you may sign up for prenatal yoga and decide to drop your book club. During pregnancy your body is making adjustments, and you will probably find that you need to make adjustments in your daily life as well.

It's essential to continue to do the things that make you happy, keep you healthy, and keep you fulfilled. If you listen to your body, you'll find ways to trim back, find shortcuts, or make substitutions that will adjust things for your pregnant needs. You need to find a balance that works for you during pregnancy. Keep in mind that your life will always be changing from this point on, as your newborn baby grows and goes through different stages. Motherhood is all about change. You need to be prepared to be flexible so that you can adjust your life to your child's needs and your needs.

To continue to do things you love during pregnancy, consider making some adjustments such as these:

- Decrease the amount of time spent on the activity, such as half an hour gardening instead of an hour.
- Take a lighter approach to the task, such as baking one batch of Christmas cookies instead of five at a time.
- Rely on conveniences, such as delivery, Internet shopping, or free carry-out service.
- Decrease the frequency, such as working late only one night a week instead of two.
- Quit sooner, such as heading home to bed at 11 p.m. instead of staying out till 1 a.m.

- Sit down more often throughout any task.
- Come prepared with food and water to any activity so you don't get hungry and thirsty.

Changing Your Perception of Who You Are

Becoming a mother doesn't have to change who you are. Still, it is likely that your pregnancy has started to create a paradigm shift inside you, and you're changing your priorities. This can be a bit nerve-wracking and uncomfortable, but it is the beginning of becoming a mother and is something that will soon come more naturally.

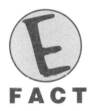

FACT

A Norwegian study found that pregnant women who were able to control their work pace (including when they took breaks) had fewer pregnancy complications, including significantly fewer instances of preeclampsia and low birth weight.

Once you become pregnant, you suddenly change from being a person who is responsible for herself to being a mother with a baby to care for. This can be a dramatic shift. It can feel frightening to suddenly give your body and your life over to someone else. You may feel a bit lost in all the changes and uncertain of who you really are anymore.

As your life starts to change and you begin to see yourself as a mother, don't lose your perception of who else you are and what else is important to you. If you have a full and active life before getting pregnant, it's unlikely that you'll be feel satisfied if you relegate the rest of your identity away so you can be "just a mother." Take the time to enjoy your newfound motherhood, though. Pregnancy is fleeting, as are the newborn days. Remind yourself to simply enjoy each day as it comes, even as you are balancing motherhood with the other parts of your life.

Now that you're adding "mom" to your list of responsibilities, it may be time to take stock of who you really are and who you really want to be. For example, some women decide that as much as they have enjoyed their career, a baby means a change to becoming an at-home mom, even if only for a few years. Other women find that the prospect of becoming a mother makes them rededicate themselves to a goal or a way of life, such as finding time to create art or becoming more spiritual. Take the time to explore who you are at this stage of your life and where you want to go from here.

Listening to Your Body

You often hear people recommending that you listen to your body during pregnancy. This may be easier said than done. Learning to hone in on the signals your body sends you is an important way to monitor your pregnancy.

The first thing to remember is that although it certainly affects your mental state, pregnancy is something that happens in your body, not your mind. You aren't in control of it, and you can't direct it. It may even seem like you are at its mercy. Because it is a physical condition, you need to learn to interpret the clues your body sends you and determine what they mean.

One important thing to remember during pregnancy is that your body really means business. When you're not pregnant, you may be able to work through fatigue, ignore thirst, bypass hunger, or push through discomfort. During pregnancy, however, you need to learn to pay heed to these signals. When you're thirsty, drink. When you're hungry, eat. Rest when you're tired. Those rules may seem obvious, but many women who have had years of experience controlling their bodies find it can be difficult to unlearn those controlling impulses.

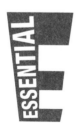

If you want to take the advice to listen to your body literally, you can purchase or rent a handheld Doppler that will allow you to listen to your baby's heartbeat. Dopplers are considered safe during pregnancy and can be a great way to bond with your baby, but they do not work well until the fourth or fifth month. Additionally, it can be hard to find the heartbeat when the baby is very active.

Fatigue is another important signal from your body. There may seem to be absolutely no reason why you should feel so tired, but what you must remember is that your body is working extremely hard building and supporting a new life. This takes vast amounts of energy. Here are some other signs that should not be ignored during pregnancy:

- **Bleeding or spotting:** While many women bleed or spot without consequences, it is always something you should be aware of and, if your health-care provider indicates, may be a sign you need to slow down. It is always a good idea to call your provider any time you have bleeding during pregnancy.
- **Pain:** Always consult your health-care provider about any pain during pregnancy, and always stop any activity that causes you pain.
- **Contractions:** While Braxton-Hicks contractions are normal in late pregnancy, painful, ongoing, or strong contractions are not, and they should be reported to your health-care provider. This kind of contraction means you need to stop whatever activity you are doing and rest. The key is that contraction sensations have a rhythm; they come and go. If you are in doubt, lie down quietly and put your hand over your uterus. If it is a contraction, you will feel the uterus become hard and then relax. If these increase in frequency, duration, and intensity, it may be preterm labor. If you are in doubt, always call your provider.
- **Swelling:** Edema, or swelling, is common in pregnancy, but it should be discussed with your health-care provider. Continued swelling is a sign you need to elevate that part of your body. Sudden and progressive swelling of the hands and face or rapid weight gain of three to five pounds may be a problem. You should call your provider and have your blood pressure checked and urine tested for protein.
- **Faintness:** Feeling dizzy or faint is something you should let your health-care provider know about, but when you experience it you need to sit or lie down. If you haven't eaten recently, do so.
- **Nausea:** This is the most common pregnancy complaint and is something you have to pay heed to. If a food makes you feel nauseous, don't eat it.

- **Discomfort:** While there's no getting around discomfort, particularly in late pregnancy, use your discomfort as a clue. If your groin muscles hurt, learn about exercises to strengthen them. If your feet hurt, put them up more often and wear more comfortable shoes.
- **Intuition:** Some women sometimes have a sense that something simply is not right with their bodies or their pregnancy. If you feel this way, don't ignore it. Tell your health-care provider, and find out if there is a basis for this warning sign.

Not Letting Pregnancy Take Over Your Life

If you're worried about getting a mommy brain, you're not alone. Many women, particularly those who are older and have careers, are loath to let themselves be defined by their growing uterus, or later by the baby they hold in their arms.

It can be a struggle to keep your pregnancy from taking over every aspect of your life—your health, your home, your job, your relationship, and more. It's important to remember that you will be a better mother if you continue to have a sense of self and continue to live a life that satisfies your own unique needs. Resting and taking care of yourself now is important, just as spending lots of time with your baby will be important once you're a mother. At the same time, refusing to let yourself be entirely defined by your parenthood status can help you keep your head screwed on straight.

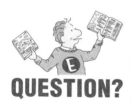

QUESTION?

Can I get a divorce while I am pregnant?
You can get a divorce while you are pregnant, but most likely the court will reserve issues of custody and child support until after the child is born, so you won't be able to completely resolve all of the issues facing you.

Sometimes it's easy to get completely caught up in the pregnancy whirlwind. You're buying maternity clothes, comparing baby monitors, deciding between cloth or disposables, rearranging your schedule, interviewing nannies, trying to understand breastfeeding basics, and more. It's okay to delve into these new and exciting things. After all, how will you ever fully understand them and come to grips with them if you don't? But at some point you may find you need to take a step back and realize that the choice between green or yellow crib bedding may not be as crucial as it can sometimes come to seem.

There are also times when you may need to remind people that there is more to you than that bump growing out in front of you. You shouldn't be sidelined from important work projects or passed over for an important role in your favorite charity's next event just because you're pregnant. Sometimes you have to make the extra effort to let people know you're still interested in being yourself and doing the things that you've always done. Often people think they are helping you by making things easier. They may not realize that you don't want your condition to be a deciding factor.

While achieving balance is so important in keeping you sane and happy, it's also important to realize that there are times when things *should* be out of balance. For example, as you get closer to your due date, more of your thoughts and energy will turn to the baby and the upcoming delivery. This is normal and good. Similarly, it is terrific if you have a very busy week at work during your second trimester and get very wrapped up in a deadline and don't think much about the pregnancy or the baby. Let your priorities naturally set themselves, and you will find that you can achieve a long-term level of balance in your life.

Dressing the Part

Baby on board? Although you definitely have a baby on board, you probably are looking for maternity clothes that fit your own sense of style and meet your daily needs. It is possible to dress like a grownup and be pregnant at the same time.

You will probably want to continue to wear your own clothes for as long as possible. You can stretch their usefulness by buying waistband expanders. There is also a product called Bella Band that allows you to wear your pants unbuttoned and partially unzipped by slipping a large fabric elastic band over it. You can buy expanders for your bras as well to give them a little longer life.

There are more choices than ever before for well-designed, quality maternity clothes. The first rule of dressing for pregnancy is to stick to what works for you. If you didn't like jumpers before you were pregnant, you're not going to like them now, so don't even consider them. Remember who you are and choose clothes that reflect that. Select colors and fabrics that appeal to your taste. Don't feel like you have to veer off into unfamiliar territory just because that's what your local maternity store is showing. You can maintain your sense of self by relying on accessories you like and that work well for you.

Some women like to purchase regular women's clothes (non-maternity) in larger sizes. This is a great way to find fashionable clothes, but they may not last to the end of your pregnancy. Your belly will grow so large by the end that normal shirts are too short in the front and normal pants will not fit over it. It is, however, a good way to shop for basics such as T-shirts, pantyhose, and other items that you can wear underneath other clothes. Additionally, some women like to wear some of their partner's clothes, at least around the house.

Shop online for the biggest selection of maternity clothes. Remember that many pregnant women find they get hot easily, especially in the last trimester, so avoid items that are very heavy. Tight clothes can be especially uncomfortable during pregnancy. Pants and skirts that are expandable are a good bet so that you can wear them smaller in the beginning and open them up to full size at the end.

Maternity clothes in general are not made to last. Most women wear items for about five months total. If you're working full-time and are trying to limit what you're spending, you're going to be wearing the same pieces over and over, so buy quality clothes that will last. If you have friends or family members with children, they may be able to lend you some of their better items, adding to your wardrobe. There is also a very brisk business of maternity clothes at secondhand stores and on eBay.

You may find you need to purchase new shoes during pregnancy. Very high heels are not recommended in pregnancy because coupled with a large uterus, they can throw your balance off.

If you experience a lot of swelling, your current shoes may no longer fit. In addition, some women find that their feet actually grow during pregnancy. This is due to the hormone relaxin, which helps relax your joints during pregnancy and can cause your feet to become longer. Foot swelling usually goes away within a month after delivery, but any foot stretching due to loose ligaments is permanent. Don't wear tight shoes. Not only do they hurt, they can also cause a lot of problems such as ingrown nails, calluses, or corns. Additionally, very uncomfortable shoes make it harder to walk and can seriously affect your balance.

Chapter 14

Commemorating Your Pregnancy and Newborn

Pregnancy and the newborn weeks are fleeting. They may seem interminable while you are going through them, but they will be over in the blink of an eye. As you hold your hands against your growing uterus or as you hold your newborn, you may wish there was a way to capture and preserve these moments. In fact, there are a multitude of ways to commemorate and preserve your pregnancy and newborn time.

Photographs

Photographs are a terrific way to capture fleeting moments. You can take photos at home yourselves, or you may choose to use a professional photographer.

Pregnancy Photos

Pregnancy photographs have become more popular in recent years. Whereas in earlier years women sought to cover it up, showing off a pregnant belly has become a style statement. If you take photos at home, you may wish to use a digital camera, which allows you to see the photos before printing them. Natural lighting is important for home photos. To help your belly show up in the photos, turn sideways and wear clothing that contrasts with the background color, or leave your belly uncovered. Some women document their pregnancies by taking one photo each month to show the changes that are happening with their bodies. This can provide an interesting retrospective. You may wish to take photos with your partner touching your belly, or with your other children in the photos. One striking photo pose is just of the mother's naked belly with the hands of loved ones on it. If you take photos at home with a digital camera, you may feel more comfortable exposing more of your body, since there is no one else around to see.

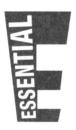

If you purchase a new camera, practice using it, downloading the photos, using the editing program, and printing photos during your pregnancy. You don't want to be in the delivery room with a brand-new camera and no experience. It is also unlikely you will have time once the baby comes to spend time learning how to crop, adjust color, and so on.

Professional pregnancy portraits can provide interesting effects. Instead of worrying about whether the photos are turning out and if you have the right kind of light, as you might when you take photos on your own at home, you can instead relax and let the photographer worry while you relax and concentrate on living the moment. Many professional pregnancy portraits are taken in a way that gives them a dreamy quality. The photographer may also use fans to cause your garments to blow or billow around you as you pose. You and your partner can both be in the photos without having to use a timer or ask anyone else to operate the camera. The photographer will most likely have backdrops and props that will enhance the photos.

You will be able to see the digital images or look at proofs before purchasing the photos. You can ask for photos in color or black and white. Look for a photographer who has taken pregnancy photos before and can show you some you like and who offers a package you consider to be affordable. For best results, schedule a photo shoot after your thirty-sixth week. Expect to pay several hundred dollars on up, depending on the length of your shoot, types of photos, and number of prints you purchase.

Baby Photos

You'll probably never use your camera as much as you do during your baby's first few weeks of life. Starting in the delivery room, you will probably begin taking hundreds of photos. Getting good baby pictures can be challenging. Natural lighting is important because flash lighting may cause shadows, or even worse, wake up the baby! Try to zoom in so that the baby takes up most of the frame. Getting down at the same level as the baby will help you take more balanced and natural-looking photos. Make sure you take photos of the baby with you, your partner, the grandparents, other children, and the special people in your lives.

Babies change so quickly that you will want to continue to take lots of photos. Snap photos of cute things she does, but also of the quiet moments, such as when she is sleeping or nursing. Make sure that you label and date all of your photos and store them in albums so that they are organized. Six months from now, you simply aren't going to remember when or where a photo was taken.

Having professional portraits taken of your baby can be a great idea. A popular shower gift is a gift certificate for a once-a-month professional photo shoot to document how the baby grows and changes that first year. When choosing a photographer, find one who works with children often. Schedule it for a time when your baby is generally calm and alert if possible, but be prepared for the worst. Make sure that you are nearby if your baby is propped up for the photo; if he starts to fall, you want to be within arm's length. Bring several outfits with you in case the baby soils one (or more).

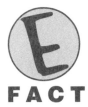

FACT

Births to mothers over 35 are on the rise, and the trend is also continuing for women at the very edge of their childbearing years. In 2003, 323 births were recorded in the U.S. to mothers who were between the age of 50 and 54, a number that is up 23 percent.

Another popular option is to take your baby to a photographer at a department or discount store, such as Wal-Mart or Sears, where you can get a lot of prints for a low price. Make an appointment if possible, and try to go during the day on a weekday. Parents of school-age children are likely to fill appointments on weekends and after school. Appointments are hard to come by in the months of November and December, when many parents are getting yearly portraits taken for use as holiday gifts.

Videos

A video allows you to have a living, moving, talking record of your pregnancy and child's early days. Videos are easy to make and fun to watch, particularly for your child when she is older.

Pregnancy

You may wish to create a video of part of your pregnancy. Recording your shower and the days before you deliver can create great memories. You may also be able to record the baby moving in your stomach during a particularly active period when the kicks are visible from the outside. Some parents like to record labor and delivery as well, but the thing to remember is that if you are relying on your partner for support during labor, there may come a time when he will need to put down the camera and focus on your needs. It can also be difficult to shoot a delivery in a modest way.

Some health-care providers and some hospitals do not permit photographing or videotaping deliveries for fear that they may be potential evidence in litigation. It is important that you discuss this with your health-care provider and know the hospital's stance on this issue.

Newborn

If you plan on videotaping your newborn, practice in advance. One of the biggest problems amateur videographers experience is camera movement, so practice getting steady shots. Film in natural light, and practice zooming. If you have editing software, you will be able to edit your tapes down and create a film of watchable length that displays your newborn.

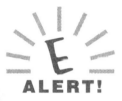

ALERT!

When printing out digital photos you took yourself, be sure to buy fade-resistant photo paper and ink. Otherwise, your photos will yellow or leech away. Save all digital images to a CD so that you have a copy of them should something happen to the photographs themselves.

When filming, it is useful to have someone on camera say the date and the age of your child at the time you are filming. When you watch the tape a year from now, you won't remember when it was taken.

Baby Books and Journals

Keeping a pregnancy journal or baby book is a great way to record events and milestones, as well as your own thoughts and reflections on pregnancy and parenthood. There are a wide variety of books you can purchase, or you can make your own.

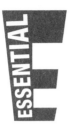

If you're a daring soul, you may be willing to let the whole world see your pregnancy and delivery or first days at home. In exchange, you receive a professionally produced and filmed tape. If this sounds intriguing, you might be interested in applying for one of several pregnancy and baby reality television shows, such as *A Baby Story* or *Bringing Home Baby*. For more information, visit *www.TLC.Discovery.com*.

Pregnancy Journals

A pregnancy journal allows you to capture your experience daily or weekly throughout your pregnancy. There are a variety of pregnancy journals you can buy that contain prompts—thought-provoking questions or suggestions—to help you figure out what to write. You can also buy a blank book, use a notebook, or create a computer file for your journal. If you write your own, here are some things you might wish to include:

- How you found out you were pregnant
- How you told your partner and other people in your life
- How you reacted to the news
- Symptoms and emotions you are going through
- Names you are considering
- The first time you felt the baby move
- Your reaction to hearing the heartbeat for the first time
- Your reaction to your ultrasound
- Your baby shower
- Plans for the nursery
- Your dreams and hopes for this baby
- Your thoughts on becoming a mother
- Your worries

Baby Books

Lots of mothers like to keep baby books that track their baby's development through the first year and possibly beyond. Many books have pages of specific questions and facts to fill out, as well as space to paste in monthly photos. Some books begin with your baby's birth, while others include some pages about pregnancy. The best way to find a baby book is to go to a bookstore and look through them so you can find one that fits your personality.

You can also make your own by using a blank book or even a computer file. Some things to include are these:

- How your labor started
- Where you gave birth and who was present
- What time your baby was born and what he weighed and measured
- Your thoughts and feelings at birth
- What coming home was like
- Baby's first visitors
- Baby's first smile
- The first time he slept through the night
- Baby's first laugh
- Visits with friends and family
- Baby gifts you received
- The first time he rolled over
- The first time he crawled
- First solid foods
- Your first kiss from the baby
- The first step
- Baby's first word
- Favorite toys
- Games you play with the baby
- Silly nicknames for the baby
- The first birthday party

Belly Casting

Pregnancy is never static; your body and your emotions are constantly changing. One thing that is certain is that pregnancy is amazing, particularly when you think about how hard your body must work to grow a human being and make room for it inside you. Because that pregnant belly will disappear (well, most of it!) when your baby is born, a lot of moms get their bellies cast as a way to preserve the beautiful shape and curves pregnancy creates so fleetingly.

A belly cast is a plaster mold of your belly and sometimes your breasts. These casts are simple to make, if a bit messy. You can do it yourself at home with a kit (available for under $40 at maternity stores and Web sites), or you can hire a local artist to do the casting for you. It's a quick process, not unlike those plaster-of-Paris art projects you may have done in art class in elementary school. First you cover your belly with Vaseline, and then you place strips of wet plaster over your belly and allow them to harden. When the cast is dry, you pull it off.

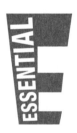

Some women like to wear special pregnancy jewelry to announce their condition and offer them inspiration throughout their nine months. You can also find jewelry specifically for home birth, fertility, and nursing. Additionally there is jewelry to commemorate a miscarriage. Once your baby is born, there are many jewelry options, including mother rings, birthstone booties, or boy/girl charms.

Once you have your cast, you can paint it or decorate it in any way you like. You can mount it to a board, or attach a wire to it so that it can hang, or you can buy a special box to store it in. No matter what you do with it, you'll find the experience fun and the cast a treasured memory of your pregnancy.

Trees

Trees are another way to commemorate your pregnancy and baby's birth. For many people a tree symbolizes life and can be a living memorial that lasts for many years.

Some families plant a deciduous tree every time a child is born in the family. The tree then becomes that child's tree to play under and climb in. Some women like to plant a tree in the same hole with the placenta so that the placenta nourishes the tree in the same way it nourished the child. The problem with planting a tree is that if you ever move, you can't take the tree with you and will have to leave it behind.

Scrapbooks

Scrapbooking has become more than a hobby and for some people is almost a way of life! You can hire a skilled scrapbooker to create a personalized scrapbook for you if you like. However, you don't have to have a professional to put together a great scrapbook of your pregnancy or about your baby.

A scrapbook is like a combination journal and photo album. It is highly visual, with lots of photos, but is also very personalized, with captions or short remembrances. You can purchase supplies specifically meant for scrapbooking, including acid-free paper, decals, decorations, backgrounds, and more. You can take scrapbook classes to learn skills and techniques, and you can also buy books about scrapbooking to give you ideas.

In addition to photos and words, you can also include items like cards, announcements, ultrasound print-outs, the name tag from the hospital bassinet, and more. Some moms start a scrapbook during pregnancy but then have a hard time finding the time to work on it after the baby comes. Buy a box where you can keep all your scrapbooking supplies and where you can toss things you want to add to the scrapbook. This way, it is all in one place whenever you can steal a few minutes to assemble it.

Other Commemorative Items

There are a variety of other ways to commemorate and preserve memories of your pregnancy and birth, as well as special remembrances of your child's birth year. Some ideas include these:

- **Wine:** Purchase wine from your child's birth year and store it (lying on its side in a cool, dark place). In Italy, this birth year wine is often drunk at the child's wedding, but you can also plan to break it out for special birthdays and occasions.
- **Coins:** You can collect one of every type of coin from your child's birth year, or you can purchase a packaged set from the U.S. Mint.
- **Newspaper or magazine:** Save the newspaper from the day of your child's birth, or a weekly news magazine from that week. These items should be stored in a sealed box in a dry place, or carefully preserved behind glass in a hanging display case.
- **Star map:** Many catalogs and Web sites will sell you a print of the way the stars appeared from your location on the night of your child's birth.
- **Quilts:** If you're done having babies, you can have your maternity clothes made into a quilt, which you use for your child or save for when he or she is trying to get pregnant, as a sort of fertility token. Instead of donating baby clothes that no longer fit, these can also be made into a quilt that is perfect for a child's bed or to save as a gift for a grandchild.
- **Wish book:** Get a blank journal and ask everyone at your baby's christening or bris to write some wishes for the baby and sign their names. Another take on this is to ask each person to give the baby a gift of a certain characteristic or quality and to write down what it is and why they chose it in a blank book.
- **Baby box:** You can buy specially decorated boxes designed to hold baby items, or you can buy a box and decorate it yourself. Store your baby's wrist and ankle bands from the hospital, as well as the cap from the nursery. You can also keep baby cards, photos, and more in this box.

- **Baby hair:** Some people like to snip a small bit of their baby's hair and keep it in a small box.
- **Hand or foot cast or impression:** You can purchase a kit to cast or make an impression of your baby's hand or foot so that you can always remember how tiny it was.
- **Framed footprints or birth certificate:** Framing a copy of your child's birth certificate or newborn footprints is a way to capture that special day.
- **Christmas ornaments:** You can purchase a "baby's first Christmas" ornament to remember your first Christmas as a mom.
- **Baby keepsake dolls:** One company (www.mybabyforever.com) will make a doll that is the same measurements as your baby at birth. The dolls come with a shirt bearing your child's name, birth date, height, and weight.

Souvenir Ultrasounds

Many parents like to have videotapes, pictures, or digital media images of the unborn baby during the pregnancy. Recently, there has been a great deal of controversy regarding commercial keepsake ultrasounds, in which the sole purpose of the ultrasound is to provide souvenir images of the baby. Individuals who are not trained in sonography often perform these. The U.S. Food and Drug Administration and the American Institute of Ultrasound in Medicine take the position that ultrasounds should only be done for medical indications and that an ultrasound should never be done for the sole purpose of providing keepsake or souvenir images of the baby. However, if you are having a medically necessary ultrasound, most centers will be happy to provide you with 2D or 3D images of the baby, since such images are routinely taken during the scan. Beware of any center that seeks to charge for or market such images.

You should also realize that most of the national organizations that set standards for obstetrical ultrasound advise physicians and hospitals against videotaping ultrasounds for fear that the tapes could potentially be used as evidence in a malpractice case. You should check with the center where you will be having your ultrasounds to find out what its rules are regarding pictures and videotaping.

Chapter 15
Labor and Delivery

At last! The moment you've been waiting for, the birth of your child, is finally here. Getting ready for labor and delivery is an exciting time. You have a lot of choices and decisions to make, but all of them will lead you to the happy result of finally becoming a mother. Labor is hard work for sure, but with a good labor coach and a good understanding with your health-care provider, you will be prepared to do that work willingly.

The Role of Your Coach

No matter how and where you give birth, having a labor coach is one recommendation that does not change. Your labor coach will offer support, comfort, encouragement, and assistance all throughout labor and delivery.

Traditionally, a woman's partner has been her labor coach, but now many women make other choices. Some women choose a close female friend, mother, sister, or other relative. Other women rely on the services of a professional doula who is trained in offering support during labor.

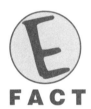

FACT

According to the CDC, the number of induced labors has doubled since 1989. Current rates show 20.5 percent of all births are induced.

Choosing someone other than your partner does not have to mean your partner is left out of the process. Most health-care providers have no problem with several people being present at a birth to offer support to the new mom. Some women designate one person as the photographer and another as their personal coach. Whatever works for you is perfectly acceptable. Some partners simply do not do well in the role of labor coach, and recognizing that and making other arrangements is sensible.

Your coach should ideally attend childbirth classes with you, so you are both prepared. Make sure you are able to reach the coach day or night as your due date approaches. You may wish to arrange for a backup coach in case your first choice is unavailable for some reason. Some hospitals require that the coach attend classes while others do not, so be sure to check into this so you can meet requirements.

Choosing a Birth Facility

When you're deciding where you would like to give birth, you may think a hospital is your only choice. In fact, you have several options to consider. Where you plan to give birth is an important component of your birth plan, and it is something you need to discuss with your health-care provider.

Birth Center

A birth center is a facility that has some medical equipment but is more comfortable and homey-feeling than a hospital. Birth centers are staffed by midwives, but they also have physicians available. These facilities often offer a wide range of birthing alternatives, such as water birth, birthing balls, birthing chairs, and other choices. Birth centers are often located next to a hospital, yet they do not have that hospital feel.

Birth center rooms are designed to look like real bedrooms. They often have kitchens and living areas for family members to make themselves comfortable in. Birth centers afford more privacy than hospitals and usually allow you to wear your own clothing.

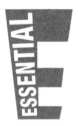

When choosing a birth center, make sure it is accredited by the Commission for the Accreditation of Birth Centers (*www.birthcenters.org*).

Birth centers have lower C-section and episiotomy rates than hospitals. While this is partially due to the approach taken in birth centers, it is also because higher-risk pregnancies are generally not accepted at birth centers because of the likelihood of complications. Epidurals are not available at most birth centers. Women who go to birth centers often receive their prenatal care at the center as well. Most insurance companies will cover the cost of a birth center birth.

When considering a birth center, ask the following questions:

- Do they accept your insurance?
- What training and certifications do attendants have?
- How many beds are available?
- Which OB or practice is on standby for complications?

- How long has the center been in operation?
- How many babies are delivered per month at the center?
- What percentage of births are transferred to the hospital?
- What kinds of pain relief are available, if any?
- If a birth is transferred to a hospital, can the midwife go with you?

Hospital

Many women feel most comfortable with a hospital birth. You have access to medical equipment if needed, and your physician or midwife can deliver the baby. When selecting a hospital, talk to your health-care provider about the level of risk you face. If you are at high risk, your health-care provider may recommend you give birth at a hospital such as a children's hospital or perinatal center, where advanced medical care is available for your newborn.

Hospitals that handle obstetrics are designated by levels one through four, with level one approved only for low-risk pregnancies and level four for the highest risk pregnancies. It is important to realize that obstetrical and neonatal care is a highly competitive business. In some instances, hospitals may attempt to market themselves as being capable of managing high-risk pregnancies when in fact the claims may be exaggerated. Health-care providers may also be partial to a particular hospital, and their decisions on the site of delivery may be based more on political than health-care considerations. If you have a high-risk pregnancy of any kind, you should ask your provider about the level of care appropriate for you. You should also ask about the hospital's capabilities. For example, a level three obstetrical hospital may have the capability to care for a problem pregnancy or premature baby, but it may not have a maternal-fetal medicine specialist or neonatologist on site twenty-four hours a day. If your baby may require pediatric specialty care, it would be best if the baby were born in a facility where that is available.

If your baby needs to be transferred after birth to a higher-level facility, you may not be able to be transferred with the baby, or if you are transferred, your insurance company may not pay for the transfer or stay at the other facility. This can be particularly problematic if you have undergone a C-section and cannot be discharged earlier. Most pregnancies can be managed in level-one or level-two facilities. Pregnancies at moderate risk (for example, premature birth over thirty weeks) can usually be managed at a level-three facility. However, the highest risk pregnancies (serious medical complications of pregnancies, birth defects, or extreme prematurity) are best managed in level-four or regional perinatal centers. Do not let community hospital politics or fancy marketing dictate the best place for your delivery.

Some physicians practice in teaching hospitals where residents and medical students are present. Many patients are concerned about having medical students and residents involved in their care. In fact, in a teaching environment where residents and medical students are well supervised, the care is actually better. However, you may have reservations about the number of individuals in the room when you are laboring and delivering or the number of people involved in your care. You should speak to your obstetrical provider about these issues during your prenatal visits. Remember, it is always your right to control these types of issues.

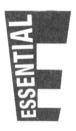

Labor is divided into three stages. The first stage, cervical dilatation, is subdivided into the latent phase (contractions without cervical dilatation) and the active phase (cervical dilatation occurs). The second stage is after full cervical dilatation, when the baby descends in the birth canal and finally delivers. The third stage is delivery of the placenta after the baby is delivered.

You should also ask your obstetrical caretaker if he has a covering caretaker(s) who will take over care should your original caretaker be on vacation, ill, or unavailable. Some physicians practice out of more than one hospital, which may create a conflict if there is a patient in more than one facility. You should also ask if there is an in-house obstetrician (or "doc in the box," as they are called). Many hospitals require or provide an obstetrician on-site twenty-four hours per day, seven days per week. The job of these obstetricians is to act in an emergency if your doctor is not available or to assist your doctor should a complicated situation come up. In many places this individual will assist your physician at a cesarean section if required.

You may also want to ask about the availability of obstetrical anesthesia coverage and epidurals in the hospital you deliver in. Though not absolutely necessary, the ideal is to have on-site twenty-four-hour anesthesia coverage for obstetrics should a problem develop. Many smaller hospitals do not have this. You should also inquire about the pediatric backup availability and credentials of those available, should the baby develop a problem in the delivery room or after birth. You should make sure that the hospital where you deliver has a transfer agreement with the regional perinatal center should the baby need additional treatment. Ask about the policy of the hospital where you are to deliver. Under what circumstances, and at what gestational age of the baby, is the mother transferred to a regional perinatal center, and which center is it? In some communities you have a choice of one or two centers. Some obstetrical care providers may make such decisions based on personal bias or convenience. You should insist upon the center that provides the highest level of care both for yourself (if you are transferred) and the baby (if the baby is transferred). Ideally, the center should have board certified neonatologists and maternal-fetal medicine specialists as well as pediatric specialists, and they should be available twenty-four hours a day, seven days a week.

Home Birth

Giving birth at home offers you the comfort of being able to labor and deliver in surroundings that are comfortable, with family present. Some families choose home birth because they want their existing children to be present. If you give birth at home, you should use a trained midwife.

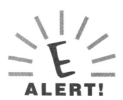

Home births are not recommended for high-risk pregnancies, women who want pain medication, or women who live more than fifty miles away from a hospital.

Home births are a controversial area in obstetrics, and most states have laws governing home deliveries. There are several considerations. First, you should remember that the purpose of the pregnancy is to have a healthy baby and mother. All other considerations must be secondary. You should also check the regulations in your state governing home births and make sure you are in compliance. Make sure that the midwife is in compliance with state regulations, is complying with safe guidelines to determine pregnancy risk, is licensed in the state where she practices, and has an obstetrical backup and plan should problems arise.

Pain-Relief Options

Many women want to know about the pain-relief options available during labor and delivery. Pain-relief options are highly evolved and can offer a lot of relief to women who choose to use them. They range from using simple breathing techniques to different types of medication. Some women decide well in advance what kind of pain-relief options they want to use. The best advice is to educate yourself about all available kinds and make your decisions as you go through labor.

Breathing and Relaxation Techniques

If you take a childbirth education class, you will learn a variety of breathing and relaxation techniques you can use during labor and delivery. The key to success with these techniques is to practice and become familiar with them in advance. The techniques are very successful in relieving pain and keeping the mother focused.

Analgesics and Narcotics

These medications provide temporary pain relief during labor through an intramuscular injection. Common medications are Demerol, Nubain, Stadol, and Sublimaze. These dull pain but do not remove it. These drugs are useful for relieving anxiety as well as pain.

Epidural

An epidural is the continuous injection of pain-relieving medications into the epidural space in the spine. The catheter is taped to your back, and the amount of medication delivered can be dialed up or down depending on your sensation or need to push. A low-dose epidural, also called a walking epidural, allows full movement while reducing pain. Pain relief with an epidural can be uneven, with more sensation on one side than the other. Pain relief is not immediate and may take time to work. More than 50 percent of all U.S. births involve epidurals. The risks involved with an epidural include low blood pressure and slowed labor.

There is considerable controversy regarding epidural anesthesia during labor, as to whether it poses risk to mother and baby, or whether it slows down labor and increases the need for vacuum or forceps delivery and C-section. In skilled hands, epidural anesthesia can be extremely beneficial and safe. As with any medical intervention during labor, the decision on its use should be individualized according to the mother, baby, and the situation. It is probably a good idea to discuss epidurals with your health-care provider. This topic is also covered in childbirth classes.

Spinal Block

A spinal block is the injection of pain-relieving medication into the spinal fluid. A spinal provides complete, immediate numbing of the middle and lower body; however, it is temporary and wears off within an hour or two. Spinals are generally reserved for C-sections. See Chapter 16 for more information about spinals.

Combination Epidural and Spinal

A combination of an epidural and spinal can provide benefits of both: the immediate relief of a spinal and the lasting effects of an epidural.

Local Injection

If you need an episiotomy, you may be given an injection at the site to numb the area. If a forceps or vacuum assisted delivery is needed, a local block is given to numb the area.

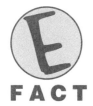

FACT

A study in the medical journal *The Lancet* found that low-dose epidurals resulted in fewer interventions during birth, with 43 percent of women being able to give birth on their own without forceps or vacuum extraction, compared to 35 percent of women who were given higher-dose epidurals. However, those with low-dose epidurals took longer to recover from birth, and their babies were more likely to need breathing assistance.

Labor Induction and Augmentation

Sometimes labor does not start naturally on its own or does not continue at a normal pace. In these instances, your health-care provider may decide to either begin labor for you or urge it along using medical procedures or medication.

Induction

If you go past your due date, experience problems that necessitate delivery, or your water breaks but labor does not begin on its own, you may need to have your labor induced. Most elective inductions of labor are performed for postdatism (usually one or two weeks past your due date), or when continuing the pregnancy may pose an unnecessary risk to the baby or mother (such as preeclampsia, maternal diabetes, or fetal growth restriction). Your health-care provider will first perform a pelvic examination to determine the ripeness of your cervix. This is determined by evaluating the softness and thickness of the cervix, effacement (thinning) of the cervix, cervical dilation (if any), and station (how high the baby is in the birth canal). A numerical score called a Bishop score is then assigned. The higher the score, the higher the likelihood of a successful induction.

There are several methods your health-care provider may choose from or combine to induce labor:

- **Stripping the membranes:** Your health-care provider separates your membranes from your uterus, which causes the release of hormones that can begin labor. This can be done at your doctor's office and can be uncomfortable.

- **Breaking your water:** Your health-care provider breaks your bag of waters (this is called an amniotomy), causing the release of hormones that will get your labor started. An amniotomy should only be performed in a hospital setting.
- **Prostaglandin analogues:** These are drugs that can be taken orally or intravaginally for both cervical ripening and induction. These drugs can cause excessive contractions (called hyperstimulation) and need to be removed should that occur. Usually, you must remain in the hospital during cervical ripening, and the process may take up to twelve hours.
- **Pitocin:** This is the hormone oxcytocin, which your health-care provider may give you intravenously to stimulate contractions. When Pitocin is used, your contractions and the baby's heart rate will be carefully monitored.
- **Cervical catheter:** Your health-care provider inserts a small catheter with an inflatable bulb on it into your cervix and expands it. This can cause the cervix to ripen and labor to start.

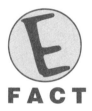

FACT

A study in the *American Journal of Obstetrics and Gynecology* found that as the mother's age increases, so does her risk of needing labor augmentation, having a prolonged labor, and needing a forceps or vacuum extraction. The same study also showed that older mothers are more likely to have babies who experience shoulder dystocia, the shoulders getting stuck during birth. Pushing the baby back in (cephalic replacement) and then performing a cesarean section is a last resort if the shoulders can't be freed.

If your health-care practitioner induces labor, but you don't give birth within forty-eight hours, she may advise you that you need a C-section. The risk of infection increases the longer you wait to deliver, especially if your water bag has broken.

Augmentation

Labor augmentation is used when your body is in labor but you aren't progressing. If your water has not broken yet, your health-care provider will likely break it for you. If that is not successful or your water has already broken, Pitocin is given by IV to increase your contractions. Because older women tend to have longer labors, they are also more likely to receive labor augmentation to attempt to move things along.

Vaginal Birth

Vaginal birth is what most mothers plan on and is considered the safest type of delivery. While the odds are that you will have an uneventful vaginal delivery, some situations are more likely to occur in older mothers. It's best to be aware of them just in case.

Prolonged Labor

Older women are more likely to have a cervix that is slower to dilate. The cervix must fully dilate and efface before you can deliver. If this process is slower than usual, your labor can go on for a long time, not only increasing fatigue but also increasing the chance of infection.

Dysfunctional or prolonged labor means the labor is not progressing at an appropriate rate. First babies tend to be slower at every stage of labor. Older women are more likely to need Pitocin augmentation, have vacuum or forceps delivery, experience prolonged labor, and have a greater chance of a C-section. The exact reason for this is not known.

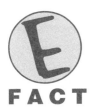

FACT

An episiotomy is a procedure in which your health-care provider cuts the area between the vagina and rectum to assist in delivering the baby and prevent tearing. Older mothers are less likely to undergo episiotomy than younger mothers. The rate for women over age 35 is about 50 percent.

Your physician can increase the odds you will deliver in a normal time frame by carefully managing your labor and using Pitocin. As a general rule, older mothers, especially those who have had more than one child, can expect to have a normal vaginal birth, but they may expect to need Pitocin to augment their labors more frequently. An important thing to keep in mind is that a longer labor is really expected for older mothers and is nothing to be overly concerned about if it happens to you. Your health-care provider will manage your care to help you deliver in a time frame that is considered normal by the medical establishment.

Breech Presentation

In normal deliveries, the head is delivered first. A breech presentation is when the baby's feet or buttocks are closest to the cervix, instead of the head. Breech births are more difficult because the legs or feet can bend and get stuck. They occur in 3 to 4 percent of all deliveries. Age increases your risk of breech birth 1.3 times for every five-year age increment. The risk at age 40 is 11 percent. The highest risk group is older mothers who are having their first baby. The exact reason for the increase in risk for older moms is not known. Some have theorized that uterine fibroids, which are more common in older women, may distort the uterine cavity.

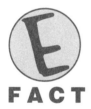

FACT

The number of women ages 40 to 45 who are giving birth is swiftly increasing. The rate for this age group doubled between 1990 and 2002. The birth rate for women age 45 to 49 has remained the same since 2000, but births in this group more than quadrupled between 1984 and 2000.

If your baby is in breech presentation, your health-care provider may try what is called an external version, in which she tries to turn the baby by applying pressure to your abdomen. This should only be attempted by an experienced health-care provider. The overall chance of success for an external version is about 70 percent, and it is usually done around thirty-seven weeks. In the United States and Canada, breech deliveries are generally not performed vaginally any longer. Many health-care providers have no experience with breech deliveries, and there is some evidence that a C-section is a safer option. Breech deliveries with twins are somewhat different. Some health-care providers will perform a vaginal delivery of a twin breech if the breech is the second twin (first twin head down, second twin breech) and the gestational age is not extremely premature.

Large-for-Gestational-Age Baby

A large-for-gestational-age (LGA) baby is one who measures over the ninetieth percentile for the gestational age of the baby, which at term is nine pounds. Large babies are common in mothers who have gestational diabetes (an increased risk for older moms), are obese, or moms who gain too much weight during pregnancy. An LGA baby can be difficult to deliver vaginally and is at a higher risk for shoulder dystocia (having shoulders that become stuck during delivery). These babies can also have low blood sugar, especially if the mother has gestational or pregestational diabetes. If a baby is still large for its age when it is six months old, it is at a higher risk for obesity. Listen to your health-care provider's recommendations for weight gain during pregnancy to try to avoid these problems.

Placenta Previa

This condition, discussed in Chapter 7, occurs when the placenta covers the cervix. A vaginal delivery is not possible in this situation. This is a condition that is usually diagnosed well before you go into labor and is usually not a surprise.

Preeclampsia and Gestational Diabetes

When these conditions are uncontrolled or at dangerous levels, your health-care provider may recommend against vaginal delivery.

Multiples

If you're carrying multiples, it is likely your health-care provider will recommend against a vaginal delivery.

Your Attitude

A 1999 study in the journal *Birth* found that older mothers seemed less likely to believe their babies' lives were in danger during labor and were happier with the way staff handled labor problems. Based on this study, it seems that older mothers tend to come away from the birth experience feeling more comfortable and secure than younger moms.

Vaginal Birth after Cesarean (VBAC)

Vaginal birth after cesarean (VBAC) has become a hotly contested topic. VBACs were once encouraged across the board. Recently, however, there have been concerns about VBAC due to highly publicized cases of uterine rupture and serious injury to both mother and baby. Because a VBAC requires an anesthesiologist to be at the ready continuously in case an emergency C-section is needed, there has been a dampening of the initial enthusiasm for the procedure, especially in level-one (low-risk) obstetrical hospitals.

The recent trend toward patient-choice C-sections also shows a declining enthusiasm on the part of many women for vaginal delivery in general, VBAC or otherwise. There has never been a randomized controlled clinical study trial comparing VBAC with repeat C-section, and it is unlikely that one will ever be done.

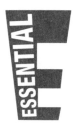

VBACs are drastically declining because of studies indicating they are not as safe as was once believed. The VBAC rate is down 67 percent since 1996 and made up only 9.2 percent of all 2004 births.

In deciding if you'd like to try a VBAC, you need to discuss the reason for your first C-section with your health-care provider. If you had a C-section previously for failure to progress in labor and this current baby seems to be about the same size, it's unlikely you will be successful with a VBAC. But a prior C-section because of breech position does not make it likely a VBAC would be unsuccessful. The most serious risk associated with VBAC is rupture of the scar from the previous C-section.

A study in the *American Journal of Obstetrics and Gynecology* found that the older a woman is, the less likely it is she will be able to successfully have a vaginal birth after a previous C-section. Among all women, about 20 to 40 percent of VBACs are unsuccessful. Those most successful with VBAC shared the following characteristics:

- Had a low-segment transverse incision with their prior section
- Have a normal-sized baby who is not in breech
- Have a pelvis large enough for the baby to fit through
- Spontaneously go into labor (are not induced)
- Have not had a C-section in the last two years
- Have not had a C-section due to a large-for-gestational-age baby

A trial of labor to see if you can progress might be something to consider, but studies show that C-sections done after failed trials of labor have higher complications than C-sections performed without any attempt at labor (that is, a scheduled C-section). You have the right to change your mind at any time during a trial of VBAC, regardless of your reasons.

In deciding whether to do a VBAC, you need to weigh the risks. A repeat C-section carries the risk of infection, a longer recovery, difficulty holding the baby, as well as all the risks of surgery, such as blood clots. A VBAC carries the risk of uterine rupture and the risk of being unsuccessful, leading to a C-section after hours of labor, which may have a higher complication rate than if it had been performed electively.

If you are induced for your VBAC, you may be at a higher risk of complications. Several recent studies have shown that the use of prostaglandin analogues for cervical ripening is associated with a higher incidence of uterine rupture for VBACs. Although Pitocin alone did not appear to increase the risk of uterine rupture, many obstetricians will no longer induce a patient with a prior C-section who wants a VBAC. However, Pitocin augmentation during labor appears to be safe in skilled hands.

Alternatives to Traditional Hospital Birth

If the idea of a traditional hospital birth does not appeal to you, a variety of options are available that offer you a choice about how to manage your pain and get through labor. It's important to note that these methods and styles of birth are not ruled out in a hospital. Many hospitals support these types of methods. You might also consider a birth center, where alternative methods of pain management are encouraged.

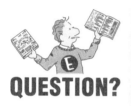

QUESTION?

How successful is a home birth likely to be?
Studies show that women who have previously had children are the most likely to have a successful home birth. One U.K. study showed that only 10 percent of women who gave birth previously were transferred to a hospital, compared to 40 percent of first-time mothers.

Hypnobirthing

Hypnobirthing is a relaxation technique that uses hypnosis to help a woman control pain during labor. The idea behind the concept is that tension increases pain. If a woman can remain relaxed through the use of hypnosis, she will feel less pain, and her labor will progress more smoothly. Hypnobirthing also incorporates other commonly used techniques, such as visualization and breathing, to create relaxation. You can work with a hypnotherapist during your pregnancy only, or you can also have the hypnotherapist accompany you to a birth center or hospital for your birth.

Water Birth

In water birth, a woman labors and delivers in a tub of warm water. The warmth of the water is soothing and is meant to ease pain. The baby is delivered under water, which is thought to be less stressful. Other advantages that are cited include reduced stress and anxiety during labor, pain relief, more rapid labor, and increased elasticity of vaginal and vulvar tissues, which makes labor easier and reduces tearing. You can purchase portable water-birth pools for use at a home birth or hospital birth.

One of the key concerns with water birth used to be the inability to monitor the labor, but there are now waterproof monitoring devices available that allow continuous or intermittent monitoring during birth. Babies who experience stress during labor due to umbilical cord compression or hypoxia (low oxygen) may gasp before the umbilical cord is cut and may suffer from water aspiration and even drowning. The warm water may keep the uterus from contracting effectively, predisposing the woman to postpartum hemorrhage. There is also a theoretical risk of maternal water embolism and breaking of the umbilical cord at birth.

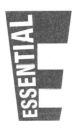

For more information about water birth, contact Water Birth International (*www.waterbirth.org*; 503-673-0026).

There is considerable disagreement in the United States about the safety and advisability of water births. The American College of Obstetrics and Gynecology has not endorsed water birth because there is a lack of data proving its safety. Most hospitals in the United States do not permit water births, so most are performed by midwives or in birthing centers. Obviously, the final word is not in on water deliveries. It is important that you inform yourself and get several opinions as well as information about outcome rates (success rates) in the center that offers the procedure.

Birth Balls

A birth ball is a large air-filled ball similar to a large exercise ball. A woman sits on the ball during labor, and the position is believed to help open the pelvis and decrease discomfort. Some hospitals have birthing balls. Most birth centers do. You can purchase a birth ball for use at a home birth or at a facility.

Positioning

Although the most common position for giving birth is lying on your back with your legs elevated, there are a variety of other positions that might feel comfortable for you or be effective. Laboring on your hands and knees can be helpful for back labor. Standing, walking, swaying, and leaning are other positions that can be helpful. Squatting can also work for some women. If you are giving birth in a hospital, you need to speak up about your preferences for delivery.

Chapter 16

Cesarean Sections (C-Sections)

Many women deliver their babies by cesarean section (C section), in fact, national averages show that C-section accounts for 29 percent of all births. C-sections are surgical procedures that are recommended when vaginal birth is not possible, labor is not progressing, the baby is in distress, multiples are being born, or the mother's health is in danger. For many women, a C-section is not an ideal birth and can feel like something of a disappointment, while other women request C-sections without a medical reason. Each woman has her own reaction to and opinion about C-sections and should be permitted to make her own choice after receiving medical advice.

C-Section Basics

While C-sections are truly a lifesaver in many instances and highly recommended in others, in general, avoiding them is the way to go if at all possible. A CDC study published in the journal *Birth* found that for mothers that were low risk, the infant mortality rate is twice as high for babies delivered by C-section than vaginally. (Note that simply being over age 35 may be considered a factor that makes you high risk.)

C-sections are surgical procedures and carry risks that include the following:

- Reaction to the anesthesia
- Blood clots
- Wound infection
- Increased bleeding
- Injuries to the bladder or bowel during the surgery
- A longer recovery time
- Increased risk of hernias due to the weakened abdominal wall
- Adhesions (Fibrin, a natural defense to tissue damage, can adhere to organs, causing twisting and pulling in the abdomen and leading to infertility, pelvic pain, and bowel obstruction.)

In addition to these risks to the mother, babies born by C-section (especially if labor has not taken place prior to the procedure) are more likely to experience temporary breathing problems after birth. This condition, called transient tachypnea, requires medical attention. The labor and delivery process normally clears fluid from the baby's lungs and releases hormones that stimulate lung activity. Missing out on labor and delivery means these things don't happen, increasing the chances of problems. Babies born by C-section may be groggy due to the medication the mother receives during the surgery. There is also a small risk of scalpel injury to the baby.

Once you have one C-section, you are much more likely to need another one in a subsequent pregnancy. This is particularly true since evidence shows repeat C-sections may be safer than VBAC for many women and due to the fact that VBAC may not be available in all hospitals. Previous C-sections increase the risk of placenta previa and placenta accreta in the pregnancies that follow. The more C-sections you have, the more scar tissue you build up, which can make future conception more difficult. Multiple C-sections also make the surgery more technically difficult, increasing the risks of prolonged surgical time, infection, and damage to other internal organs such as the bladder or the bowel.

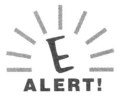

ALERT!

If you have a C-section, ask your physician to use adhesion barriers. These barriers, which are not common in C-sections although they are for other abdominal surgeries, prevent the growth of adhesions that can cause many problems. Another request to make is for suturing of the peritoneum, the membrane that covers the internal organs. Often in C-sections it is left to close on its own, but a recent study showed suturing it prevents adhesions.

Another risk of C-sections is that your baby may be born too early. If your C-section is not preceded by natural labor and is instead scheduled or follows an induced labor, your baby may be slightly premature if the calculations used for your due date were not accurate. Preterm babies face the risk of jaundice, breathing problems, feeding difficulties, and an inability to properly regulate body temperature. Generally, though, if your pregnancy is accurately dated, performing an elective C-section prior to labor can be done from thirty-nine weeks on without concern about fetal lung immaturity. If you need a C-section sooner, or if the dating of the pregnancy is in question, an amniocentesis can check the baby's lung maturity. Women who are HIV-positive and who are having a C-section to prevent transmission of HIV to the newborn may have an elective delivery at thirty-eight weeks, so that the C-section is performed before labor begins. The risk of the baby having respiratory problems is relatively low under these circumstances.

Patient-Choice C-Sections

Patient-choice C-sections (those done based on a patient's request, and not for any medical reason) have seemingly become popular in recent years. Many celebrities schedule them, and according to Health Grades, an independent health-care ratings agency, the number of women choosing patient-choice C-sections rose by 36.6 percent between 2001 and 2003. However, these procedures are not nearly as popular as the media has portrayed them. One study showed that approximately 96 percent of women preferred a spontaneous vaginal delivery. Of the 4 percent who said they would prefer a C-section, the majority either had some type of risk factor that they thought made C-section safer for the baby or had a bad experience with a prior vaginal delivery.

Women who choose patient choice sections do so for a variety of reasons:

- Fear of the pain or embarrassment of labor and delivery
- A need to exactly plan the birth date for work or personal reasons
- A belief that avoiding delivery will prevent bladder control problems later in life
- A belief that delivery will change their vagina permanently, making sex different or less pleasurable
- A belief that delivery negatively impacts the pelvic floor muscle tone
- Fear that problems during delivery will harm the baby, causing problems such as cerebral palsy

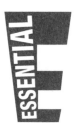

The American College of Obstetricians and Gynecologists (ACOG) has issued a formal policy on patient-choice C-sections, saying it is ethical if it is in the best interest of the patient both physically and emotionally. Because of this policy, many physicians are willing to perform patient-choice C-sections.

Some of these reasons are valid, and some are not as valid. Some women are simply not able to face labor and delivery for a variety of reasons, and having the option of a C-section is important for them. Each woman has to make a decision about what is right for her personally, and she should be permitted to do so. Some women need to be able to plan an exact birth date due to pressing career, family, or personal reasons, and they should be supported in their need to do so. It is also true that a vaginal delivery does stretch out vaginal tissue and that it can never be exactly as it was before. The vagina is designed to stretch, though, and any change is minimal. Most women find that they have normal, satisfying sex lives after a vaginal birth.

The information about pelvic floor changes causing a loss of muscle tone or leading to incontinence is conflicting. While there is evidence that vaginal birth can lead to these problems, the primary culprit is probably carrying a pregnancy. The weight of a baby on your pelvic floor for so many months is more likely to cause changes that lead to muscle tone changes or future incontinence.

While problems can occur during vaginal birth that can impact the baby, most problems are present before delivery, including increasing evidence that cerebral palsy is not caused by birth trauma. Some women see birth as a risky situation. While it is true that labor and delivery can be unpredictable, a competent physician can manage just about anything that happens. A C-section is not without risks either, so neither option is considered entirely risk-free.

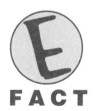

FACT

A 2003 Gallup poll showed that one-third of female OB/GYNs interviewed said they would perform a patient-choice C-section if a patient asked.

Acceptance

No matter how you come to have a C-section, ultimately you have to accept the fact that you've had one and come to terms with it. Whether your baby exits your body through your vagina or through an incision in your uterus, you have still given birth and still have grown and nurtured a human being inside your body. You are a mother either way. The type of birth you have is a small part of your baby's history and does not mean you are any less of a woman or mother.

It is important to remember that both vaginal birth and C-section birth require stamina, courage, and commitment. Whichever you end up going through, you have accomplished something to be proud of.

Reasons for C-Sections

Unquestionably, there are situations in which C-sections are the best and safest choice for both the mother and baby. If your health-care provider recommends a C-section for you, take her advice seriously.

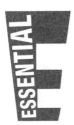

For information about C-sections, see the Maternity Center Association's downloadable pamphlet on making the choice (online at *www .MaternityWise.org* and *www.ICAN-online.org*).

A C-section might be recommended to you for a variety of reasons, including the following:

- Previous C-sections or abdominal surgeries
- A baby that is too large to be safely delivered vaginally
- Placenta previa (the placenta covering the cervix)
- Placental abruption (the placenta pulling away from the wall of the uterus)
- Failure to progress in labor, or labor that is too slow
- An infection such as genital herpes or HIV
- Gestational diabetes or preeclampsia (C-section not necessary but in some cases is recommended)
- Multiples
- Breech position
- Umbilical cord prolapse (the umbilical cord slips down into the vagina, possibly cutting off oxygen supply to the baby)
- Shoulder dystocia (the baby's head is delivered but the shoulders are stuck under the mother's pubic bone).

- Prior third- or fourth-degree tear in a previous delivery (if the muscle around the anus or the rectum tears, a subsequent vaginal birth can increase the risk of bowel problems)
- Nonreassuring fetal status, previously called fetal distress (a slowing of baby's heart rate, indicating a problem)

In some situations, an emergency C-section is necessary and there is no time for your physician to discuss the options and risks with you. In this instance, follow the medical advice you receive and let your trained professionals do what they are trained to do. There are other instances when you have time to agree to a C-section and ask questions.

How to Decrease Your Chances

Because a C-section is major surgery and carries risks, most women wish to avoid having one if possible. It's not always possible to avoid a section, but there are things you can do to reduce your odds.

Age

First of all, you have to realize that your odds of a C-section are simply higher because of your age. According to the March of Dimes, about 40 percent of women over age 35 will have a C-section. While this figure is high, it does not mean that you will need a C-section. If you actively work to avoid one, you may improve your odds. Keep in mind that your physician is also aware of these statistics. While most physicians do not prejudge a woman's ability to give birth solely based on age, some may be less inclined to work with you to avoid a C-section. Talk to your doctor about what you can do to reduce the chances of a C-section, and make clear your desire to avoid one.

Be Educated

Read and educate yourself about pregnancy, labor, birth, and C-sections so that you will understand whatever happens and will be prepared to deal with it. Arming yourself with knowledge is also likely to reduce anxiety and tension, and it may help you relax more during labor, leading to a successful outcome.

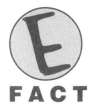

FACT

Women who have C-sections are less likely to be successful at breast-feeding. This may be in part to discomfort from the incision, making positioning difficult.

Take a childbirth education class. If this is your first child, it is an essential step to take. You will not only learn about pregnancy, labor, and delivery, but also about breathing and relaxation techniques that will help you cope with labor more successfully. If you had a previous C-section and want to try for a VBAC, ask about a VBAC class.

Stay Healthy

Staying healthy during your pregnancy and following your health-care provider's recommendations are key. Eating a healthy, well-balanced diet and exercising will keep your body in good condition and help you prepare for labor. Also, not gaining excessive amounts of weight, or following your diet strictly if you have gestational diabetes, will reduce the risks of having an oversized baby that can't be delivered vaginally.

Stay Home

Once you go into labor, follow your health-care provider's instructions about when to contact him and when to go to the hospital. Remaining at home as long as possible during the first stages of labor can help you remain calm and relaxed and reduce the risk of medical intervention.

Epidurals and Labor Augmentation

Some studies show that epidurals slow down labor. If you are very concerned about this, you may wish to use alternative relaxation techniques during your labor. If your baby is overdue, the risk of the epidural slowing things is outweighed by the benefit of getting the baby delivered before size becomes an issue.

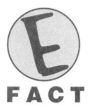

FACT

When your baby is born, he will be evaluated using an Apgar score. The baby is observed at one minute and five minutes after birth. Each of the following factors is rated on a scale of zero to two: heart rate, breathing, activity and muscle tone, the grimace response, and skin appearance. Studies have shown that babies of older mothers score just as well on the Apgar test as those of younger mothers.

Having your labor induced or augmented also increases your chances of having a C-section, although this is most likely the result of the way your labor is progressing rather than the fault of the medication. The risk of needing a C-section from an induction increases if the cervix is not ripe. The use of cervical ripening agents reduces this risk. If the induction fails after two days, most patients will opt for a C-section rather than going home to wait for labor to start naturally. The take-home message is that unnecessary inductions (not medically or obstetrically indicated) should be avoided.

Ultrasounds

Medical opinion used to be that doing a late third-trimester ultrasound could help decide if the baby was large and if induction would reduce the risk of a C-section or shoulder dystocia. However, it has been shown that the risk of shoulder dystocia actually increased in women who were induced in these situations, and the risk of C-section also increased. It is now not recommended that nondiabetics have an ultrasound to help make this determination. For diabetic pregnancies, however, it is legitimate to base delivery decisions on ultrasound-estimated fetal weight.

Stay Mobile

Move around during labor. Remaining in bed on your back does not help your body. Standing, walking, squatting, swaying, and other movements may help move your labor along.

What to Expect

Unless you've already had one, a C-section can seem a little scary, particularly because the entire procedure is completely out of your control, yet it happens right in front of you. Understanding what to expect can make the process easier and more comfortable.

Preparation

Before your C-section, if it is not an emergency, you will talk with your health-care provider about the decision to have a C-section. This is the time to ask any last-minute questions or express any concerns. You will talk to the anesthesiologist, who will get a medical history from you and discuss your anesthesia options. If you do not already have one, an IV will be started in your hand so that medication can be administered. You will be taken into a surgical delivery room. Your abdomen will be washed and shaved. The anesthesiologist will administer your medication. A catheter will be inserted into your bladder. Sheets will be set up to block your view of the procedure. Your partner and/or coach will be allowed to join you.

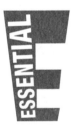

If you will be having, or think you may be having a C-section, you may want to join C-Section Support, an online group for moms who have had or are about to have a C-section (online at *http://groups.msn.com/CSectionSupport*).

The Surgery

Your physician will make an incision into your abdomen. There are several types of incisions. The most common and most preferred is the low-segment transverse incision, or bikini cut. The physician cuts through your abdomen and then through your uterus. It only takes about three minutes from the time of incision to the time of delivery. You will feel nothing, other than some tugging. The physician will then reach in or push on your stomach to get the baby out. The baby will be suctioned (to clear the nose and mouth), and your incision will be closed. The skin incision is usually closed using surgical staples or with subcuticular sutures (sutures under the skin). The subcuticular sutures are more cosmetically appealing just after the surgery, and there is nothing to remove. However, staples are faster to place, and removal causes minimal discomfort. The wound looks the same with either method within several weeks after the surgery. Rarely, a drain may be placed temporarily inside the wound, usually attached to a small plastic bulb or circular cylinder for draining the wound.

Throughout the procedure, you will be surrounded by nurses and physicians who are there to care for you. If you feel uncomfortable in any way, let them know. After your baby is born, you will be able to see her, and your coach or partner will be able to hold her.

After your surgery, you will go to the recovery room, and your baby will go to the nursery for evaluation. Once your condition is stabilized, you'll be moved to a regular room, and your baby will join you.

Preventing Problems

The risk of uterine and abdominal wound infections is very high following a C-section, especially if labor occurred or membranes ruptured prior to the procedure. Preventive antibiotics are given as a single IV dose after the baby has been delivered to prevent problems.

Pregnant women are at higher risk for blood clots in general. When a blood clot forms in a large vein in the body, it is called deep vein thrombosis (DVT). If part of this blood clot breaks off and embolizes (moves) to the lung, it is a pulmonary embolism (PE). PE and DVT are called thromboembolic disease or complications. Women who have C-sections are at higher risk for these complications especially if they are older, obese, have varicose veins, or smoke. Women who have a C-section after labor or who have a uterine infection at the time of delivery are also at greater risk.

Thromboembolism after C-section is prevented using a small dose of blood thinner (Heparin) or sequential pneumatic compression stockings (stockings that gently squeeze your legs). Heparin must be given prior to the C-section and continued for a time period after the surgery. The sequential stockings are placed around the calves (they look and feel a lot like blood pressure cuffs) prior to the surgery and are connected to a machine that inflates and deflates the cuff. This pumps the veins in the lower extremities. There is some evidence that an epidural can help prevent deep vein thrombosis.

Another problem that a C-section can lead to is the need for a blood transfusion. For a routine C-section, the risk of needing a blood transfusion is relatively low. However, in certain circumstances such as placenta previa, especially in the presence of suspected placenta accreta (where the placenta invades the wall of the uterus, more common after a prior C-section), the need for a blood transfusion is relatively high.

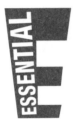

In most hospitals, a sample of blood is taken from the umbilical cord after delivery and sent for analysis of the pH level of the baby's blood. This shows the baby's oxygen levels at the time of delivery and can be used to determine if problems occurred prior to or during labor and whether the baby may need extra attention. Talk to your pediatrician about these test results.

Autologous blood transfusion, in which the pregnant woman donates her own blood in advance of the surgery, is an option. There was controversy at one time regarding pregnant women doing this, but it appears to be safe if performed to certain guidelines. Having a friend or relative donate (if they are compatible) is also possible; however, it is not always possible to know for sure if the individual who you have chosen to donate may in fact be a risky donor. Another possibility is called Cell Saver. This procedure collects blood from the patient's own pelvis or abdomen, recycles it, and transfuses the blood back to the patient. However, there is a significant risk of amniotic fluid spilling into the abdomen, mixing with the blood, and causing an embolism. Finally, the hormone erythropoietin (available as Eprex, NeoRcormon, or Aranesp) can be given by injection for several weeks prior to the surgery. This drug stimulates the bone marrow to make more blood and can raise the concentration of hemoglobin. Both erythropoietin and Cell Saver are usually acceptable to patients who are Jehovah's Witnesses or oppose blood transfusions.

Pain Relief

One of your primary concerns about C-sections is likely to be pain relief. You will be able to remain completely pain-free during a C-section and will have an anesthesiologist who is completely devoted to making sure you remain comfortable.

Epidural

An epidural provides pain relief through a catheter that is inserted into the epidural space in the spine, and left in. One of the biggest benefits of an epidural is that it can be used for vaginal delivery or C-section. Because the pain relief can be increased and controlled as needed, it works for both types of deliveries. If you come to the hospital and intend to give birth vaginally, you may choose to have an epidural for pain relief. If the decision is made that you need a C-section, you won't need another needle in your back; instead, the amount of your epidural is simply increased. In most circumstances you must stick with the epidural for the surgery and cannot have a spinal after an epidural has been placed. If general anesthesia is necessary (for an emergency C-section), it is safe after an epidural.

The main drawback with an epidural for C-sections is that it may not provide complete pain relief. There may be areas that are not completely numbed. An important benefit of the epidural for C-sections is that it can be left in place after the surgery and used for post-surgical pain relief.

Spinal

Spinals are administered by an anesthesiologist through an injection directly into the spinal fluid. They take effect immediately, but they only last sixty to ninety minutes and cannot be readministered during the surgery. If for some reason the surgery does not go as planned and cannot be completed in that time frame, general anesthesia would be necessary.

The spinal completely numbs your mid- to lower body. The numbness may spread to the chest area so that you can no longer feel yourself breathing; however, you do not stop breathing. This sensation can be a bit alarming, but it is in no way dangerous. There is a rare condition called a high spinal in which the muscles of respiration are paralyzed. The patient would then be given general anesthesia.

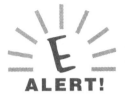

ALERT!

During spinals and epidurals, you can experience nausea and may begin to vomit. This generally occurs after the baby is delivered. The anesthesiologist will administer medications to help with this, and the feeling usually passes quickly. Report any feelings of nausea right away.

General Anesthesia

General anesthesia is most often used for C-sections when there is an emergency and your physician has to get the baby out quickly. The other types of anesthesia take time to administer, but general anesthesia can be administered very, very quickly. If you have general anesthesia you will sleep through the entire birth and won't feel anything. Some women experience nausea after awakening from general anesthesia, but this is reduced with the use of antiemetic drugs.

Chapter 17
Recovery

Once you're finally a new mom, you will mostly likely be floating on air, wondering at the beauty of your new baby. However, this is a time when you must also focus on yourself and your own recovery from the birth. It takes time to recover from the actual birth process, just as it takes time to adjust to caring for the new little person who has joined your family.

Recovery from Vaginal Birth

Although birth is a natural process, it can sure take a lot out of a person. When recovering from vaginal birth, it is important to give yourself time and not to expect an overnight recovery. Remember that it took nine months to carry your pregnancy and that recovery is something you should view as an ongoing process.

If you deliver in a hospital, you will mostly likely have a two-day hospital stay. If you deliver at a birth center, you will most likely go home the same day. If you deliver at home, you will want to take time to rest and recover there. You will likely experience soreness and discomfort from the birth as well as fatigue. If you had an episiotomy or have tears, you will need to care for the stitches or tears as directed by your health-care provider, which will begin with ice packs in the delivery room. You'll need to wash your hands before and after using the bathroom and avoid touching the perineal area as much as possible. A clean peri-pad is applied (front to back to avoid bacterial contamination of the perineum). Warm sitz baths offer considerable relief, as does lying on your side and sitting on a pillow or inflatable cushion. Often sprays or ointments are offered for pain relief, and oral pain medication is also offered. If a third- (torn anal sphincter) or fourth-degree (torn rectum) tear has occurred and was repaired, stool softeners will be important. If you've had stitches, it may take a few months to fully recover from them.

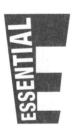

If you're anxious to begin an exercise program after birth, it's important that you talk to your physician. After a vaginal birth, you should wait four to six weeks. After a C-section you may be advised to wait up to ten weeks, although stretching is acceptable immediately after birth. The key to beginning an exercise program is to start gradually.

About a third of women who deliver vaginally develop hemorrhoids, and many others experience constipation. Make sure you get enough fiber in your diet and drink enough fluids in the days after the birth. Your health-care provider may prescribe a stool softener. If you have difficultly urinating after birth, you may need a catheter at first.

After giving birth, you will have heavy discharge, called lochia. This can contain clots and will continue for weeks. You may feel what are known as afterpains, as your uterus shrinks back to its normal size, which can feel stronger when breastfeeding. This is normal. Your breasts will feel sore as your milk comes in. Recovery from a vaginal birth is generally thought to take about a month, but every woman's experience is different.

Recovery from C-Section

Recovering from a C-section is similar in some ways to recovery from vaginal birth, since your body is recovering from carrying a baby; however, because you had surgery, recovery is more complicated. A hospital stay for a C-section averages three to four days, and total recovery takes about six weeks.

Just as with vaginal birth, you will have a heavy discharge for weeks after the birth, afterpains, sore breasts, constipation, and possibly hemorrhoids, as well as trouble urinating on your own. If you went through labor, your recovery may be more difficult because you're recovering from the surgery and the hard work of labor.

After a C-section, you will experience pain and discomfort around your incision when you try to move around. It can be helpful to hold a pillow against your abdomen when coughing, walking, or laughing to help reduce discomfort. It is important to get out of bed and move after the surgery, either the same day or the next day, to help prevent blood clots. The incision may burn and itch as it starts to heal, and this can last for several weeks. It is essential that you follow your doctor's instructions for caring for the incision, which will probably include keeping the wound clean and dry. It is likely you will have numbness at the site of the incision that in some cases can be permanent.

The hospital personnel will encourage you to do some breathing exercises to help clear your lungs after surgery. Digestive functioning may take some time to get moving again, and it's not uncommon to experience uncomfortable trapped gas. Because it takes time for digestion to resume normally, you will be placed on a liquid diet until you are able to pass gas. Getting up and moving around can help increase digestive functioning.

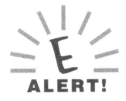

ALERT!

Contact your health-care provider immediately if you have any of the following in the weeks after birth: you experience a fever; soak more than one sanitary pad per hour; have increased redness around an incision or have pus; feel pain, swelling, or tenderness in your legs; experience coughing; have nausea; have unpleasant-smelling vaginal discharge; experience increased pain; or you have redness on your breasts or cracked or bleeding nipples.

You'll be advised to avoid stairs and heavy lifting until your incision heals. You will probably be advised not to drive a car for about two weeks or until you are able to make sudden movements.

Your physician will most likely prescribe pain-relief medication for you after the surgery, which may at first be delivered intravenously (often by a pump you can control) and then switched to pills. Speak up about your pain, and don't be afraid to ask for more pain relief if you need it.

Postpartum Depression

Approximately 80 percent of new moms experience the baby blues—feelings of sadness, anxiousness, or helplessness. This is a natural reaction not only to your new situation but also to the rapid hormonal changes (rapid decreases of estrogen and progesterone) that are taking place inside your body. While the baby blues pass for most women within days or a week, postpartum depression is a more serious and longer-lasting situation.

Postpartum depression sounds similar to the baby blues, with women experiencing some of the same emotions. The difference is that postpartum depression interferes with your ability to function and handle everyday activities over a long period of time. Symptoms of postpartum depression include the following:

- Lack of energy or motivation
- Feelings of sadness, hopelessness, and being overwhelmed
- Frequent crying
- Overeating or undereating
- Feelings of worthlessness or guilt
- Inability to focus or concentrate, remember things, or make decisions
- Sleep dysfunction—too much or not enough sleep
- Headaches, chest pains, hyperventilation, or heart palpitations
- Lack of interest in things that usually bring you pleasure or interest
- Social withdrawal

Many of the above symptoms by themselves are completely normal. It's likely you may be very tired and need to sleep, or you may have trouble sleeping with a newborn in the house—that's nothing abnormal. Additionally, if you're recovering from a difficult birth, you might not feel like seeing a lot of people, or you might find your whole life turned upside down by having a baby. These feelings are normal. But when many of them are combined, and they interfere with your ability to live your life and to simply move forward, you need to see your physician.

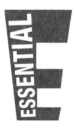

Postpartum psychosis is a rare and extreme version of postpartum depression that affects about one or two out of every 1,000 women. It includes hallucinations, delusions, and obsessive thoughts about the baby. It usually appears within the first six weeks after birth and requires immediate treatment.

If you experience symptoms that worry you or are making your life difficult, it is essential that you tell someone about them. Talk to your partner as well as to your health-care practitioner. There is nothing to be embarrassed about, and none of it is your fault or due to any deficiency on your part. Seeing a therapist or taking antidepressants, or both, have proven to be very effective in treating postpartum depression. Women who already suffer from severe depression or manic-depressive illness are at extremely high risk for postpartum depression; it is important that such women keep in close contact with their mental health-care provider in the immediate weeks following delivery.

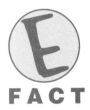

FACT

Your health-care provider will let you know when you can begin to have sexual relations again, usually about four to six weeks after birth. Generally you'll be given the all-clear at your postpartum checkup. Remember to have patience with your body. It has done a lot of work and may not respond in the same old ways.

In addition to talking to your health-care provider, rest as much as you can. Get others to help you around the house and with the baby, and talk about your feelings to anyone who will listen. Keep busy with activities and people, and remember that you have just gone through a very significant life-changing event. You can't expect to bounce back immediately.

Coping with Sleep Deprivation

Babies need round-the-clock care. Coupled with the physical recovery from childbirth, this can make a person very, very tired. Coping with sleep deprivation can be challenging.

Many parents are geared up for all-nighters when they bring a baby home, but often the first few weeks are not that difficult, since many babies do a lot of sleeping. Just when you think things are working out quite well, your newborn may surprise you with increased nighttime activity. Whether you're walking the floors when your baby first comes home or a few weeks later, it can be exhausting and frustrating.

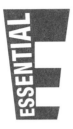

More and more women are seeking out help not only with the baby but for their own recovery after a birth. Postpartum doulas are trained assistants who come to your home and help with baby care and more by meeting your needs and those of your household, including light cleaning, cooking, errands, as well as comfort measures for the recovering mom.

Try these tips to help you manage the difficult weeks and months when you feel like a walking zombie:

- **Sleep when the baby sleeps.** It's old advice, but it works. There are times when you must get things done; if possible, try to do them with the baby awake, so you can sleep when he does.
- **Get serious about sleep.** Pull the shades, wear a sleep mask, turn off the TV, get in bed, turn off the phone, and do everything you can to maximize your sleep.
- **Get help.** Everyone needs a break. Ask your partner, friends, family, or hired help to assist you. Even if you are breastfeeding, someone else can give the baby a bottle of expressed milk at night, or at the very least, change and soothe her.
- **Relax your standards.** Because you're going to need to get some sleep during the day, you're just not going to be able to do it all, all the time. Cut back on work, reduce your household cleaning requirements, or use paper plates to make things easier.
- **Avoid tired traps.** Sometimes when you're exhausted it's easy to overeat, park yourself in front of the TV instead of going to bed, or skip exercise. None of these things will make you feel better; in fact, they'll just make you feel worse. Drinking caffeine to stay awake will only make it more difficult to fall asleep when the opportunity presents itself.

If you're heading back to work, getting enough sleep at night can be crucial. Share the burden with your partner if at all possible. If necessary, schedule a fifteen-minute catnap for yourself to get through the day. Going to bed early in the evening will also help ensure you get enough sleep.

Nursing or Bottlefeeding

How you feed your baby is a choice that is purely up to you. Your pediatrician can discuss the benefits of each method with you, but you will need to decide on the best choice for your family. Whichever you choose, adapting to this new way of providing nutrients is bound to be an experience.

Breastfeeding

Breastfeeding has many benefits for mother and baby. The American Academy of Pediatrics recommends breastfeeding exclusively for the first six months and continuing to breastfeed until age one year. Some studies indicate breastfeeding raises a baby's IQ and improves his immune system. Babies who breastfeed have lower incidences of diabetes, asthma, and sudden infant death syndrome (SIDS). Breastfeeding is also thought to enhance bonding between mother and baby. Breastfeeding is cost-free, unless you purchase a pump, and is also preparation-free. Breastfeeding reduces a mother's risk of ovarian and breast cancers and is related to a decreased risk of osteoporosis.

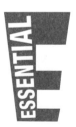

For help and support with nursing, contact the La Leche League (online at *www.lalecheleague.org*). They offer local support groups as well as publications and information.

Breastfeeding, however, requires a commitment that can be difficult. You're always on call, either to your baby or your pump, and you have to keep your milk supply going with frequent nursing or pumping. Some women find breastfeeding painful or are uncomfortable breastfeeding around others, which imposes limitations. Others find it difficult to work and nurse, requiring pumping breaks.

If you are breastfeeding, you require an additional 500 calories a day; some women find it easy to lose weight while breastfeeding. It is also important to continue to take a vitamin with iron at this time. Some women continue to take their prenatal vitamins. While breastfeeding it is important to avoid alcohol, many over-the-counter and prescription drugs, and smoking. Women who are HIV-positive should not breastfeed.

Formula

Formula is an excellent alternative to breast milk. It is not difficult to prepare and very portable if you use individual cans or powder. Formula allows anyone to feed the baby and can offer more freedom to a busy mom.

Formula does require a lot of washing of bottles and nipples and requires more work for a middle-of-the-night feeding. It's easier to overfeed a formula-fed baby since the tendency is to try to get the baby to finish the bottle rather than let the baby end the feeding when she is full.

Discovering Yourself As a Mother

Becoming a mother is a life-altering experience. Your entire perspective shifts, and suddenly you have a baby who is your number-one priority. Discovering yourself as a mother is an amazing experience, but it can also be challenging.

Some women come into motherhood determined to conquer it like a career. If you've waited a long time to have a baby, it can be easy to feel you've got to make the most of it or that you must let your baby become your world. There are many types of mothers and endless appropriate ways to parent. Reading parenting books can help you get a feel for what style of parenting you are most comfortable with, and it can open your eyes to options you may not have considered or thought possible.

The most important thing you can do as a mother is listen to yourself and follow your instincts. You might believe you don't have parenting instincts, but you do have instincts about how you want to live your life, what kind of family you want to have, and your general approach to life. Listen to these instincts and let them guide you as you make parenting decisions. More than anything else, it is important that as you parent, you remain true to yourself. If it doesn't feel right to you, don't do it, even if all the books and your mother and your best friend tell you otherwise.

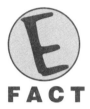

FACT

The American Academy of Pediatrics recommends that mothers and babies sleep "in proximity to each other" to encourage breastfeeding. This stops short of endorsing co-sleeping or family beds. Some physicians believe family beds are dangerous and can lead to suffocation or increased risk of SIDS. Others believe that if done safely, it can enhance bonding and make breastfeeding easier.

All mothers make mistakes, and you will, too. You can't avoid it, and you shouldn't waste your time worrying about it. Mothering is a challenging undertaking that requires twenty-four-hour management. It is your flaws that will give your family its unique character. You can probably think of things your parents did that you swear you'll never do to your child. It's terrific that you already have some ideas about what you want to avoid, but you can be sure that you will make other mistakes and errors in judgment along the way. In the scheme of things, they won't matter because your baby will have a devoted and loving mother who has good intentions.

Your Relationship As Parents

Having a baby is a major change, and it can be a big change for your relationship with your partner as well. Learning to love each other as parents can be wonderfully rewarding, though, and working together to raise a child can bring you closer.

If this is your first child, you are undergoing a major change from being a couple to being a family. Previously, you and your partner decided things together and focused on each other. Now, suddenly, a new demanding person wants all of your time and energy. Instead of focusing on each other, you and your partner now are focusing together on your baby. After a while, you may miss the time and attention you used to be able to give each other. To keep your relationship as adults alive, plan time to spend alone together. You don't have to get a sitter and go out to a restaurant; just sitting and talking about adult things for half an hour while the baby sleeps can be enough.

Learning to parent together takes time and patience. It takes time for your parenting styles to emerge, and the most important thing to remember is that you are both learning as you go. You may not always agree about how to parent, and that's okay. You probably have parents who employed different parenting styles, and so you come to parenthood with a different set of expectations and experiences.

Weight Loss

Losing your pregnancy weight is probably something on your mind after you give birth. When you give birth, you will lose approximately ten pounds and look as if you are about six months pregnant. Weight loss is a gradual process and should be taken slowly. Your goal should be to lose no more than one or two pounds per week, with about a half a pound a week being a reasonable goal. It can take years to lose pregnancy weight.

The most important thing you can do about losing weight after you have a baby is to be realistic. Weight loss by itself is difficult, but it is even more difficult when you are caring for a baby. Eating a healthy diet should be your primary concern. You won't have the energy motherhood requires if you aren't getting enough nutrients. Exercise is key in weight loss, and though you may find you simply can't exercise as much or in the same way that you used to, any kind of exercise you can fit into your life will be good for you.

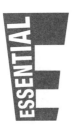

Use the post-pregnancy weight loss calculator at Babycenter.com (*www .babycenter.com/calculators/postpartumweight*) to calculate exactly how many calories you should eat per day to lose weight after having a baby. The calculator is personalized based on height, weight, activity level, and whether you are breastfeeding.

It took nine months to gain your pregnancy weight, and it is not reasonable to expect to lose it in a short period of time. Pregnancy changes your body. After you have your baby, you may desperately want your old body back, but it is something that can't happen in a healthy way overnight.

Chapter 18

Working and Parenting

If your career was an important part of your life before you became pregnant, it is likely that you are concerned about how you are going to balance your work and your new family. Each woman finds balance in her own way. Day care or a nanny may be the solution you seek. For other women, changing work hours is a solution. Other moms choose to stay home with their children. No matter what decision you make, be sure it is the one that is right for you and your family. One thing to remember is that babies grow. What is right for you now might change in a few years.

Deciding When to Return to Work

Heading back to work after you've had a baby can be challenging. Not only is it difficult to decide on the right time, the adjustment itself can be hard. When you go back to work may be dependent on how much paid and unpaid leave you have. For many women, that consideration makes the decision for them. You might, however, decide you're ready to go back sooner, or you might feel you need more time.

Making the Decision

You may not have a choice in when you return to work. If your paid leave is set to expire at a certain date and your family needs the income, the choice is most likely made for you. If you're out on an unpaid leave, deciding when to return may be more dependent on your feelings. If you've agreed to a set date to return to work, you may feel obligated to stick to it, but if you have more unpaid leave at your disposal, it really is up to you when you will return.

When deciding when to return to work, the first thing you should do is talk to your health-care provider and find out when she feels it is safe for you to return to work. Your next consideration is your mental and emotional state. When will you feel ready to direct your attention to work, and when will you feel comfortable leaving your baby? This answer is different for every woman, and no matter what your answer, it is right.

Another important consideration is child care. If you are unable to line up child care, returning to work will be nearly impossible. Start to make child-care plans as far in advance as possible. Some mothers get on the waiting list at a day-care center when they learn they are pregnant.

Going Back Sooner

If you want to go back to work sooner than you originally planned, it's likely your employer will be happy to see you back. If you have not used all of your federal Family and Medical Leave Act (FMLA) time or state family medical leave time, you may be able to use what remains to ease your transition back to work by working shorter days or fewer days per week in the beginning. You may also decide to save some of those days should your child need care within the same twelve-month period.

Postponing Your Return

You have to make plans for your leave while you're pregnant, and as a result you end up doing so without knowing what motherhood is going to be like. You can't know how it will truly affect you and your desire to return to work. If you feel you aren't ready to go back to work when your leave time ends, have a conversation with your boss about the options available to you. You may be able to work part-time for a while, do some work from home, or you may receive assurances that whenever you're ready to come back, they will have a place for you.

Making the Transition

No matter when you return to work, the transition is huge. Your entire life has changed since the last time you were at work. Leaving the baby can be difficult emotionally as well as physically, due to fatigue and if you are breastfeeding. To make the transition easier, follow these tips:

- **Make a gradual transition.** Try to slowly get back to your work schedule instead of suddenly being back at your desk full-time.
- **Have a few dry runs.** Take your child to day care or have the nanny come before the day you go back to work. You want to work out any problems in advance so that when you do go back, you can feel confident your baby is well cared for. If you're going to be pumping at work, start your pumping schedule while at home.
- **Don't expect too much of yourself.** You won't be able to get right back in the groove, and it will take you time to adjust. You can't expect everything to be as it was, given that your life has changed so significantly.
- **Expect to be emotional.** Leaving your baby can be hard. Don't try to keep it all bottled up inside. It can be hard to redirect your focus on work when you're thinking only of your baby. Forgive yourself for the distraction you feel.

- **Plan to check in on the baby.** Call the sitter or day care, or stop in during your lunch hour. Touching base in the middle of your day will help you relax and know your baby is doing just fine.

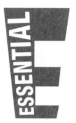

Many states have laws about breastfeeding, including the right to pump at work. You can check your state laws about breastfeeding at *www.ncsl.org/programs/health/breast50.htm*.

Day Care

Day care is an excellent child-care option. Most centers will accept infants over six weeks of age. It's important to research day-care centers during your pregnancy as many have waiting lists for infants. You also don't want to make this decision at the last minute, when you're under pressure to return to work soon. You need time to visit the centers and evaluate them before making a decision.

Important Considerations

When choosing a day-care center, it's important to listen to your instincts about the facility and the people who work there. In addition, there are other practical considerations to ask about and look for when you are evaluating a center:

- **Costs:** Ask about weekly rates, hourly rates, and additional charges for extra hours. Some centers have registration fees and yearly supply fees as well. Ask if you are expected to supply snacks or supplies.
- **Sanitary measures:** Find out what their policy is. Toys and equipment should be cleaned regularly, and after a toy is mouthed it needs to be cleaned. The diaper-changing area must be cleaned after each use, and staff should wear gloves and/or wash hands each time.
- **Sleeping arrangements:** Ask if all infants must follow the same schedule of naps or whether babies can sleep as needed. Make sure each

baby has a separate crib. If the center provides linens, they should be washed daily.

- **Hours of operation:** Some centers only accept full-time enrollment, so ask about part-time if that is your interest. Learn the hours they are open, as well as holiday schedules and closings due to weather. Ask about vacation and sick day policies as well.
- **Safety standards:** All equipment should meet safety standards and be checked for safety regularly. Safety also includes windows and doors, which can be hazardous if windows are floor-length, doors are made of glass, or mini-blinds are used. Bookcases should be bolted to the walls, electrical outlets covered, and outdoor play areas fenced. Smoke alarms, emergency plans, and compliance with fire codes are essential.
- **Feeding:** Learn if breastfeeding is encouraged and if mothers are welcome to come feed their babies. Milk and formula should be labeled and stored in the refrigerator. Parents should supply bottles and be responsible for washing them at home. Learn if babies are fed on a schedule or on demand.
- **Staff information:** Make sure all staff is trained in first aid, that they can provide references, and that their backgrounds have been checked. They should also have current immunizations. A director should be on the premises at all times.
- **Age separation:** Children should be grouped by age, with infants cared for in a room separate from other children.
- **Sick policy:** Learn what symptoms indicate your child should be kept home. Immunization requirements should meet the ones created by the American Academy of Pediatrics. Learn if there is a nurse or physician on call.
- **Parent involvement:** Some centers require parents to participate a certain number of hours a month. At the very least, parent involvement should be encouraged and welcomed.
- **Contract:** Ask to see the contract in advance, and look for liability waivers in it that say the center has no liability at all for your child.

In-Home Day-Care Centers

Many women run day-care centers out of their homes. Often they are home caring for their own children and agree to care for several other children at the same time. These centers feel more home-like. However, there are likely to be fewer resources and not as much backup available.

When evaluating a home day care, learn where in the home the children will be cared for and if it is childproofed and separate from the rest of the home. Determine how the provider will ensure equal treatment among her own children and your child. If there are other staff members, get information about their qualifications, training, and background.

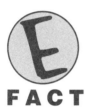

FACT

In-home day-care centers are regulated and licensed by the state. If the center does not have a license, it is operating illegally. Ask to see all state documents, and call the state licensing board to determine if any complaints have been filed against the center. You can find state regulations at *www.daycare.com/states.html*.

Relative Care

Having a relative care for your baby can be convenient and inexpensive. You also have the peace of mind of knowing that someone who loves your baby is providing care.

In the beginning, when your baby is small, it may make more sense for your relative to care for the baby at your home. After all, all the supplies and equipment needed are there. Eventually though, you may agree to take the baby to the relative's home.

When you work out the arrangement, have a frank talk about pay. Many grandparents don't want to be paid, but other relatives might expect payment. Don't forget to consider compensation for travel and expenses such as diapers and formula. If this is an older relative, talk about current recommendations, such as putting babies to sleep on their backs, not starting solid foods until six months, and other "modern" child-care concepts.

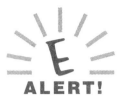

Be sure that the relative's home is completely childproofed. You also need to make sure that all baby equipment used at the home, such as cribs and high chairs, meet current safety recommendations. For example, some relatives like to use old cribs whose bars are too far apart to be safe.

Hiring a Nanny

A nanny can be a great child-care choice, as she will work in your home and care solely for your child. However, hiring a nanny is more expensive than a day-care center and presents some tax difficulties.

Agency Nannies

When you hire an agency nanny, you contract with an agency that provides you with a nanny. The agency screens the nannies, handles all payroll taxes, and can readily supply another nanny should one not work out. When working with an agency, get details on their screening process and minimum qualifications for nannies. Make sure you have the right to turn down a candidate they offer. Ask if the agency does unannounced spot checks on nannies in their employ. Be sure to get references for the agency.

Au Pairs

An au pair is a child-care worker, similar to a nanny, who is often a young foreign woman in the United States on a visa. She lives with your family and provides full-time child care in exchange for room and board, transportation, and a small stipend. To find an au pair, you need to work with an au pair agency. Ask how the girls are chosen, how good their English must be, how many hours they are expected to work, and how long they are placed with you. Get references for the agency.

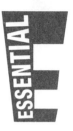

No matter what kind of child-care arrangements you make, it is essential that you create a backup plan. This is necessary for days when your child is too sick to go to day care, the sitter cancels, or you have to stay at work late and can't pick up your child on time.

Sitters

If you hire someone yourself to act as a nanny or a babysitter in your home, make sure you get references and check them carefully. Find out how experienced she is with infants. Set clear guidelines for what you expect her to do in addition to child care, if anything. Make sure you stop in unexpectedly once in a while to see how things are going. You will be responsible for payroll taxes for the nanny or sitter.

Changing Your Schedule

Some women find that when they return to work, they need to change their work schedules. There are a variety of options available to you if you're considering this.

Changing Your Hours

If you work shifts, you may consider changing your shift to allow you to spend more time with your baby during the day. If you work in a business where there are no set business hours, you may be able to change your work hours to better fit your family's needs, but only if it meets with your supervisor's approval.

Changing Your Job Arrangement

As discussed in Chapter 10, two other options available to you are job-sharing and flex-time. Job-sharing allows you and another person to share the duties and hours of one job. Flex-time allows you to work the same amount of hours, but at flexible times. Both of these options are very family friendly and may allow you needed flexibility, but they require the approval of your supervisor.

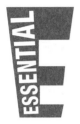

Working Mother magazine publishes a list each year of the most family-friendly companies to work for. You can find information about it on their Web site, online at *www.workingmother.com*.

Some women find that having a baby is an impetus for a career change, such as going part-time for a few years, taking a different position that may be more family-friendly, or changing companies to one that is more family focused. Other women find that having a baby creates a shift in their priorities. They may stay in the same job with the same hours, but they find that their baby has become the most important thing.

Working at Home

Working from home is an option a lot of women dream about, but is not without its benefits and detriments.

Working from home is a delicate balance. On the one hand, you get to spend more time with your child, spend less money on child care, commuting, wardrobe, and office expenses. However, it can be quite difficult to actually get any work done if you have no child-care help. Additionally, many women miss seeing colleagues, getting out of the house, and having more time to themselves. Some women experience a sudden dissonance, going from working in a job they and others see as important to being stuck in the house all day, working in sweats, and having no visibility.

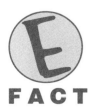

According to the U.S. Census Bureau, 53 percent of married mothers with children one year of age or under are in the workforce. One half of mothers return to work within six months of their child's birth.

If you want to work from home, there are several options to consider. You could work out an arrangement with your current employer that allows you to work from home and still be an employee. This kind of arrangement is usually not completely work from home and often requires some face-time in the office. Another option is to work for yourself, either in your previous line of work, by opening a home business, or by doing some kind of freelance or consulting work. No matter what your plans, it is usually a good idea to arrange some kind of child care so that you can have time to actually work.

Becoming an At-Home Mom

Many women choose to stay at home with their babies, whether they are permanently leaving their careers behind or simply putting them on hold for a few years. The U.S. Census shows that 48 percent of children under the age of two are cared for solely by a parent. On average, women stay home with their children 2.2 years before returning to work.

Staying at home with your baby means the loss of your income, but it also can mean a large savings. When choosing whether to stay at home, you need to weigh the loss of your salary and benefits against these savings:

- Work/career clothing and shoe costs
- Dry cleaning expenses
- Commuter costs (gas and car maintenance or public transportation)
- Work lunches, coffee, and other snacks
- Office gifts and parties
- Business expenses (such as briefcase, cell phone, and appointment book)
- Child-care costs

In addition to these hard savings, there are a variety of other ways that staying home cuts your expenses. You will be less likely to spend money on convenience items such as prepared food, takeout, delivery services, and so on, because you will have more time and won't need to rely on these services as often. Being a stay-at-home mom may mean you'll have the time and energy to do things such as cook and bake, clean your own home, make gifts, become a comparison shopper, do your own laundry, or devise low-cost children's activities, all of which can offer significant savings.

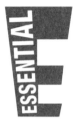

For help and support in your role as a stay-at-home mom, contact Family and Home Network (*www.familyandhome.org*) and the National Association of At-Home Mothers (*www.athomemothers.com*).

Staying at home is not all craft projects and time to read magazines. It is full-time hard work. First of all, make sure that both you and your partner value what you're doing. Raising a child is an admirable task. If you didn't do it, you'd need to pay someone else. Make time for yourself, whether it means hiring a sitter occasionally or getting your partner to assume child-care duties. Set realistic goals for yourself as a stay-at-home mom. For example, if you've never liked to cook, it's unlikely you'll start to enjoy it now. It is very difficult to be a full-time mom, full-time cleaning lady, full-time chef, full-time partner, and more, so don't expect more of yourself than is possible.

At-Home Dads

In 14 percent of families where the mother works, the father stays home with the children. In many families, having an at-home parent is important. The choice about who will stay home is often made by comparing income, benefits, and hours, as well as considering who feels most passionately about his or her career and who is most able to take time out from the workforce. Dads do just as good a job as moms, and it is a choice each family must make for themselves.

Sharing the Parenting Burden

You and your partner created your baby together, and you probably hope to raise her together as well. Working together as parents is the only way to ensure that you can both pursue your own individual career dreams or life goals.

While it is fairly common for women to assume most child-care responsibilities, you and your partner can work things out in any way that feels right to the two of you. It can be nearly impossible for a woman to return to a full-time job and bear the entire child-care burden when she is home, including evenings and through the night. You've got to sleep sometime. You and your partner might work out a schedule that divides up child-care tasks, such as designated nights for each of you to care for the baby or planning who will handle bath time each evening so the other person can have some personal time. Planning individual outings is another way you and your partner can share responsibilities. Designate a certain night of the week as individual outing night and alternate whose turn it is to go.

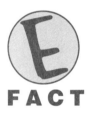

FACT

Only one out of three women who qualify for pregnancy leave in the state of California take the leave, according to *Maternal and Child Health Journal*.

Sharing the parenting load is very much about a state of mind. If you see yourself as solely responsible for your baby, assume your partner doesn't know how to care for the baby, or act as if he doesn't do things right, you're going to create a situation in which the main burden of parenting will fall upon your shoulders. It's likely you'll share things more equally if you enter parenting with the mindset that you are both parents and although you might do things in different ways, you are equally qualified and equally responsible for your child. It is extremely beneficial for children to have both parents involved in their upbringing, so parenting together is a smart choice.

Chapter 19
Life As an Older Mom

Being a mom is a wonderful new experience that adds an entirely different enriching perspective to your life and your experiences. Being an older mom does pose some unique challenges. Women over age 35 who have babies usually already have very full and busy lives. You may have other children, older parents who depend upon you, as well as a full slate of interests, activities, friends, and responsibilities that are important to you. Learning to balance all of these things together with a new baby takes some practice, but it is ultimately extremely rewarding.

Enjoying Every Moment

One thing you will find is that babies grow very, very quickly. There are moments and days that may seem interminable when you are living them (colic, crying, messy diapers, sleeplessness, and so on), but when you look back on things, you will be amazed at how very quickly it has all gone. Reminding yourself now and then to enjoy these times will help you stay focused and centered.

No matter what your situation, your child is a precious gift. It can still be easy to lose yourself in the daily craziness of new motherhood. Feeding time, when your baby is quiet and happy and very close to you, is a good opportunity to reflect on your child and new motherhood.

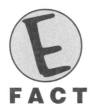

Older mothers are substantially more likely to breastfeed. Of mothers age 30 and over, 44 percent breastfeed, compared to only 30 percent of these ages 20 to 29.

If you think you won't have any more children, you might feel sad to watch your child grow up. The nice thing about children is that as much as you love them at one stage, you are sure to love them at least as much at the next stage and the next stage. They are an ongoing source of inspiration and joy, no matter how old they get. And no matter what stage your child has reached, you will always be her mother and there to see it all firsthand.

Avoiding Becoming Over the Top

If you have waited a long time to have a baby, or had to try very hard to get pregnant, your child may seem like quite a miracle to you. Some parents in this situation go overboard coddling their children. While your joy and relief is natural, you have to find a way to keep it from becoming your only focus. Being overprotective, overly indulgent, or too permissive won't express your gratitude and love and instead is likely to cause problems for your child.

Readjusting Priorities and Expectations

Becoming a mother adds more to your to-do list. If you had a marriage and a job and a home and a pet before, now you've still got those things, but you've also got a wonderful baby you want to devote a lot of time to. Something has to give. You can't continue to do everything you did before, to the same standards and requirements, while also fitting a baby into your life.

This is the time in your life to make changes and simplify, if you can. This is not to say you can't excel, do things well, and achieve amazing things. Motherhood doesn't have to crimp your style, but it does mean you have to choose what is important to you and focus on those things first.

A lot of women always expect too much of themselves. They feel they have to keep a perfect house, excel in their career, have wonderful friendships, do community or charity work, have a size-zero toned body, create romance, cook beautiful meals, and more. This is hard enough to do on an ordinary day, but on a day when you're trying to care for a baby and adjust to new motherhood, it is simply impossible. You must choose where you're going to excel and accept that some other things simply are not going to get done, at least not to the level you might have preferred pre-baby.

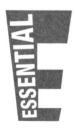

While most pregnancy magazines are geared to moms under age 35, there is a magazine exclusively for older moms: *Plum: The Complete Pregnancy Guide for Women 35+* is published twice a year by the American College of Obstetricians and Gynecologists. You can find copies at your health-care provider's office, or you can order them online at *www .plummagazine.com.*

If you don't reduce your priorities and instead move on full steam ahead, certain that you can and will do it all, you will likely become exhausted, frustrated, overwhelmed, and possibly depressed. Instead of succeeding at doing everything well, you will likely find you're doing everything, but none of it well at all. Organizing your priorities does not have to mean that you'll decide to be a great mom and everything else will go to pot. Instead, it means reducing your standards and expectations, and accepting that things may not get done as soon or as well as you want.

An important skill is learning to delegate. Delegate tasks to your partner, parents, friends, older children, coworkers, and anyone else you can. Carrying the entire burden by yourself is too much. If you get other people to help you do things, it will still all get done without wearing you out.

Sandwich Generation

The sandwich generation is made up of people who are the primary caregiver for their own children and their aging parents. Sandwich-generation caregivers tend to have careers, further complicating the balancing act they are managing.

If you are a member of the sandwich generation, you may find that you spend a lot of your time focusing on the people you are caring for and not yourself. One important key to surviving this kind of situation is to have backup. You must have someone available to care for your child should you need to take a parent to the hospital, and someone must be available to step in and help your parent should your entire household come down with strep throat.

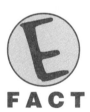

FACT

Of people providing care to aging parents, 60 percent are women. It is estimated there are 26 million women in the United States with children under the age of 18 who provide care to aging parents.

Getting and staying organized is another lifesaver. Schedules, calendars, lists, carefully filed information, and general orderliness of the "stuff" around you will help you stay sane, find what you need, and keep things together. Here are some other tips to help you keep all the balls in the air:

- **Prioritize.** When making a decision about which fire to put out first, always triage. Weigh the needs involved, and deal with those that are most pressing at that moment.

- **Rely on other people.** You can't do all of this alone, and you shouldn't have to. Your siblings and other relatives, or perhaps a visiting nurse, can help with elder care. Your partner, sitter, or older children can help with the baby and the house. Your assistant and coworkers can carry the weight of certain responsibilities at work. If you aren't comfortable delegating, now is the time to learn. It's the best way to get things done.
- **Set reasonable expectations.** As discussed earlier in this chapter, you can't do everything perfectly. There isn't time in the day. You've got to give yourself some slack some of the time.
- **Get professional advice.** You follow your pediatrician's advice for your child, so you should get and follow professional advice when it comes to caring for your parent. A gerontologist is a physician who specializes in treating older patients and can help you arrange care and make decisions.
- **Remember you have family leave options.** Under the Family Medical Leave Act (FMLA) you can take unpaid leave to care for an ill family member, including an aging parent or a child. This type of leave can be very important at crucial points in your life.

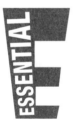

If you work less than full-time, you're not alone. An Institute for Women's Policy Research study found that half of working moms work part-time jobs, work part of the year, or work in a part-time job that does not last all year. The average workweek for year-round working moms is thirty-eight hours.

If your parents are aging but do not yet require careful care, you are pre-sandwich generation, and you can probably plan on becoming a true sandwich generation member within a few years. To make things easier should your parents require more care in the future, you should get organized now. Living closer to your parents makes things exponentially easier.

Finding Time for You

No matter how you choose to parent, it is important that motherhood be but one of the many definitions of who you are. Motherhood can feel quite all-consuming in the beginning, and it does take a lot of energy to just be a mom. But the other parts of you are important as well, and you should try not to lose them. You may not have a lot of time to pursue them, but they must remain part of your life in some way.

Although part of what you're doing is rearranging your life so that you have time for a baby, that doesn't mean you have to lose all your "me time." In fact, making time for things that are important only to you and benefit only you are very important in helping you feel like a real person and maintaining your self esteem. You can't nurture another person if you don't nurture yourself first.

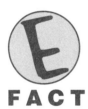

FACT

Older mothers are more likely to stay together with the child's father, so these children are more likely to be raised in a two-parent home.

In order to be a good mother, you must first be a fulfilled and complete person. In order to achieve that, you must do things for yourself. You may be pressed for time, but there are small ways to recharge your batteries:

- Get a sitter so you can get a mani-pedi or a haircut.
- Do something fun on your lunch hour, like a quick shopping trip or lunch at a nice restaurant.
- Buy yourself a treat to enjoy while the baby is asleep.
- Skip doing the dishes one night and watch a DVD instead.
- Use a bottle of expressed milk so you can have some wine.
- Arrange for your partner to get up with the baby one weekend morning so you can sleep in.
- Read a book while nursing or feeding the baby.
- Take a bath while your partner or your mom watches the baby.

- Schedule a night out with your friends.
- Take the baby for a long walk during nap time.
- Keep a sketchpad or notebook handy and draw or write while the baby is occupied.
- Surf or shop online while rocking the baby side to side on your swivel desk chair.

Finding Time for Your Partner

After time for yourself, time for your partner is often the next thing to get lost in the busy days of motherhood. Making time to connect with your partner and share things together is an important way to keep your relationship alive.

Once you become parents, it can be hard to find time for just the two of you. For many months, you may feel as if you're just trying to survive and get enough sleep. Once you've settled into your routine, finding time for the two of you can be complicated, involving babysitters, feeding schedules, naps, and considerations of what time you have to get up in the mornings.

Here are some ways you can find time for each other:

- Schedule time together at home when you'll simply talk, snuggle, or watch a DVD together. Planning at-home dates means much less pressure than trying to go out and doesn't involve a babysitter.
- Talk on the phone and use e-mail and IM. You don't have to be in the same room to communicate and feel close to each other.
- Support each other's interests. If you don't allow each other time to do the things that inspire and interest each of you, when you are together, you will have nothing to talk about other than the baby.
- Plan to have sex. It may be the last thing you're interested in, but if you do it, the ingrained reactions will kick in. You will rediscover how nice it can be, and it will help you feel closer to each other.
- Rely on relatives. It might feel like too much to book a sitter so you can go out to dinner. Not only is it complicated, but it can be expensive too if you're living on reduced income due to maternity leave. Grandparents, aunts, uncles, and other relatives adore having time

with the baby, and the baby deserves to get to know them, so rely on them some of the time. It's a win/win situation for everyone involved.

• Connect while the baby is occupied. If she's happily drooling away in her bouncy seat, use this as a few minutes to talk about something important.

• Make chores work for you. Washing the dishes together is a great time to just kid around or talk about something that's been on your mind. Link your minds while your hands are occupied.

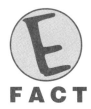

FACT

A twenty-year study performed by the RAND Institute on Education and Training found that children of older mothers had higher test scores than children of younger mothers.

It is not uncommon for your partner to feel a bit left out in the early months of your baby's life. Particularly if you are breastfeeding, you are using a lot of your time and energy to care for your baby. Even if you aren't breastfeeding, becoming a mother is a very physical commitment. Many women feel too tired for sex, and some partners feel they are somehow left out of the very intimate mother-baby circle.

In addition to finding time for you and your partner to connect as a couple, it is also important to find ways for your partner and the baby to have time together. It can sometimes be tempting as a mom to feel like you're the only one who knows how to care for the baby; if you spend all day with the baby, it is likely you will be more skilled, at least initially. However, your partner deserves a chance to parent, too, and that means walking out of the room and letting him change the diaper, do the feeding, or soothe the baby, even if he doesn't do it quite the way you would. He needs time and space to learn his own parenting techniques, and he needs your support to do that.

Finding Time for Your Other Children

If this isn't your first child, you're already well versed in what to expect as a new mom, but you may find adjusting to being a mom of more than one to be a challenge. You have the same number of hours in the day, but you now must divide them among your children. You also have to learn how to deal with siblings. Even if you already have two or more children, adding another one changes the dynamic of the family.

Other Young Children

If you are raising other young children, the demands on your time are very physical. Chasing after a toddler while caring for an infant can be challenging. The hardest part about caring for young children is that they aren't able to understand that you can only do one thing at a time and are not able to be patient. Caring for two little ones means learning to do a lot of things with one hand. Wearing your baby in a sling can be a good solution a lot of the time. A double stroller is another good answer, since it allows you to become mobile. You also can multitask during feedings; read a book, do a puzzle, color, or do another quiet, stationary activity with your older child while you are feeding the baby.

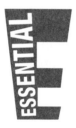

If you're finding it difficult to adjust to being a mother and find that sometimes it simply seems too difficult of a life change, you're not alone. A 2003 study conducted in Australia found that first-time mothers who were over age 35 reported that adjusting to motherhood was extremely challenging.

Young children are often jealous of the very close physical contact you share with the baby. They may want to try to nurse or push the baby out of the way. Using feeding time as cuddle time for all of you is an effective solution, and young children are so active it's unlikely they'll stay put through an entire feeding.

Older Children

If you have a family that includes children who are older and have now added an infant to the family, the logistics of mothering can be hard at times. For example, you need to nurse, but your older child needs to be driven to soccer practice. Or your baby needs to nap, but your child has friends over and they are keeping the baby awake. These and other scenarios can truly put a mother to the test.

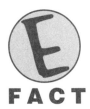

FACT

Half of U.S. presidents were firstborn children. Many newscasters and talk-shows hosts are firstborns as well.

The best way to approach a family of diversely aged children is to help everyone understand that needs must be balanced. Nobody gets what he wants all the time, and compromise is necessary. Older children are often enamored with a baby for longer than younger children. Your older child may be more understanding about the seemingly unreasonable demands a baby makes on you and on the family, but it does help to explain to the older kids that the baby doesn't mean to be demanding and annoying.

Older children can be a definite blessing because they can help you in significant ways. For example, an eight-year-old could be trusted to stay in the family room and watch the baby for a few minutes while you go to the bathroom, can answer the phone while you're feeding the baby, or can hold the baby for a few minutes while you pay for groceries.

As you already know, your older children need you in a different way than younger children do. Older kids need your mental and emotional attention more than your physical hands-on attention. The key to offering this kind of attention is affirming their needs—you know that they need to talk to you, need help with homework, or need you to help fix their hair—and pinpointing when you will be able to do that. If you're walking a screaming baby, you cannot give your older children your undivided attention. Ask them to be patient with you and the baby, and let them know that as soon as you physically can, you will turn your attention to their needs. The good thing about older children is that a little bit of attention can go a long way, so be sure to offer quality attention when you are truly focusing.

Stepchildren

If your partner has children from a previous relationship, you may wonder how bringing your own baby into the mix will work out. Your new baby is the product of both families and is in a way a unifying factor—although your stepchildren definitely may not see the baby that way! Before the baby is born, reassure your stepchildren, just as you would children of your own, that the baby will not take away their role or importance in the family. Stress how much it means to you that the baby will belong to all of you and will be related to all of you.

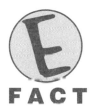

FACT

Fifty percent of U.S. families are stepfamilies, according to the Stepfamily Foundation, and in fact the U.S. Census predicted there will soon be more stepfamilies than traditional two-parent families.

Don't be surprised if your stepchildren, just like biological children, at first resent the baby or are slow to warm up to him. It takes time to build a relationship, and it takes time to build trust in a family's love. Encourage your stepchildren to help care for the baby. Stress how grateful you are for their help, and point out how much the baby enjoys their company.

If your stepchildren do not live with you, they may be angry or jealous that this new child gets to live with their father all the time, whereas they are only able to visit. Help them know that your home is their home just as much as it is the baby's home.

Finding Support

Parenting can feel like a lonely occupation. You spend much of your time with a demanding, fickle, uncommunicative little person who, though the love of your life, can certainly put you through the wringer at times. This a time in your life when you need support. Just having someone else to talk to who knows what you are going through can make you feel immeasurably better.

Friends and Family

Friends and family can provide important support. Your own mother or mother-in-law can be a great support person for you. She's been through it all and has made it to the other side. Although a lot of things about childrearing have changed over the years, the basic skills have not.

Sisters, sisters-in-law, and other close relatives are another great source of support. Since they're closer to your age, they are more likely to understand about today's parenting challenges. Friends with children are important. Not only are they going through the same things, they are able to offer advice without the added baggage or expectations that sometimes comes with advice from family. Forging close relationships with friends or relatives with children close in age to yours can give you a sense of community and let you rely on each other for things such as babysitting, play dates, and shoulders to cry on.

Mothers' Groups

Reaching out and finding a local mothers' group is a great way to make new friends who are mothers and who may be experiencing a lot of what you are. Mothers' groups can be formally organized or casually drawn together. You can find listings of formal clubs in church newsletters, regional family magazines, on community bulletin boards, and through word of mouth. Some mothers' clubs form among those attending the same childbirth education class or prenatal exercise class.

Other groups come together in less organized ways. You might strike up a conversation with a mom at day care and eventually meet her and another friend of hers for coffee. Moms in your neighborhood or on your block might become friends.

While moms' groups can be a true lifeline, there can be some difficulties navigating them. If you're joining an established group, you may feel like an outsider until you get to know everyone. There may be people in the group you simply don't click with, or as your children grow, you might find that the kids don't get along very well. Ultimately you have to do what is right for you and your child in these kinds of situations.

Online Support

While having a friend who can hug you and baby-sit for you is a great thing, it is possible to make friends whom you don't know in person. You can now find any kind of specialized support group online that you could ever dream of. Some women join due-date clubs while they're pregnant and converse online with other women due in the same month they are. Many of these groups last for years, as the women support each other through the many stages their children go through.

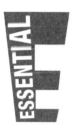

Babycenter.com has bulletin boards for pregnant moms over 35 and over 40 at *www.babycenter.com/boards/bcuspreggen* and *www.babycen ter.com/boards/bcusparentage*. Clubmom.com has a work/life balance board for moms at *www.clubmom.com/jforum/forums/show/49.page*.

Online groups can be a convenient way to make friends since you can read and send messages at any time of day. It's important to be careful and not offer personal information (such as addresses, phone numbers, and so on) online unless you really and truly know someone very well.

Chapter 20

Your Health after Pregnancy

Once your pregnancy is over, you shouldn't stop taking care of yourself. There are many health concerns you should be aware of after you are over 35 and as you age. The key to being able to care for your child is staying healthy yourself. It is sometimes easy to put your own health last on your list of priorities as you raise a family and live your life. However, staying healthy should be a priority in your life.

20

Birth Control

Many women think that because they are older and/or because they had a difficult time getting pregnant, birth control is not necessary. As long as you are not menopausal, birth control should be something you take seriously. Many older women fail to do so and because of this, a study by the Alan Guttmacher Institute showed that more than half of pregnancies in women over age 40 were unintended.

When choosing a method of birth control, you should consult with your health-care provider and choose the method best suited to you, based on your health and your comfort level with the various methods.

The Pill

If you have always used the birth control pill as your form of birth control, now that you are over age 35, your health-care provider may recommend using a different form of birth control. This is particularly true if you smoke, have high blood pressure, or have a history of blood clots or cancer. The pill is considered safe for most women over age 35 who do not meet these criteria. The pill is considered 99-percent effective, but it offers no protection against STDs. You may want to consider one of the new types of pills, such as Seasonale or Seasonique, that allow you to go three months without having a period.

Barrier Methods

Barrier methods of birth control include the condom, diaphragm, cervical cap, shield, and sponge. The male condom is 84 to 98 percent effective at preventing pregnancy and has the added benefit of reducing the risk of transmission of most STDs. The female condom is 79 to 95 percent effective in preventing pregnancy.

The diaphragm, cervical cap, and shield are devices you insert to cover the cervix. They are used with spermicide to block sperm. These barrier methods must be left in place for six to eight hours after intercourse to be effective, and are between 68 and 94 percent effective, depending on the method. The cervical cap is less effective in women who have had a child. If you use a diaphragm, you need to be refitted after you have a baby because the size of your cervix may change. These methods do not protect against STDs.

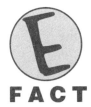

FACT

The birth control pill is the most popular type of birth control for women of all ages. The second most popular is female sterilization, or tubal ligation.

The sponge is a cervical covering that comes pre-filled with spermicide. It is not as effective in women who have had a child (only 84 to 91 percent). Like other cervical methods of birth control, it has to be left in place after intercourse for twenty-four hours to be effective. It offers no protection against STDs.

IUD

The IUD, or intrauterine device, may be either a copper T-shaped device or a device containing the hormone progesterone that is placed in your uterus. The copper IUD prevents sperm from traveling to your fallopian tubes. The progesterone-containing IUD releases hormones that thicken your cervical mucous, preventing sperm from entering the uterus and preventing implantation. IUDs are 98 percent effective in preventing pregnancy, but they offer no protection against STDs.

Hormone-Releasing Methods

There are three methods of hormone delivery that don't involve taking pills. Depo-Provera is an injection of hormones you receive every three months. Lunelle is a monthly injection of hormones. The Patch (Ortho Evra) is an adhesive patch you leave in place on your skin for three weeks at a time and that releases hormones into your body to prevent ovulation. Nuva Ring is a ring that is placed in the vagina for three weeks at a time and releases hormones that prevent ovulation. These methods are 99 percent effective. They offer no protection against STDs.

Sterilization

Vasectomy, for men, and tubal ligation, for women, are surgical methods of permanently preventing pregnancy. In vasectomy, the vas deferens, the tube that carries sperm from the testicles, is cut, preventing the ejaculation of sperm. In tubal ligation, the fallopian tubes, which carry eggs from the ovaries to the uterus, are closed or shut so that eggs cannot travel through them.

The tubal ligation procedure is performed through a laparoscope. If the tubal ligation is performed postpartum (usually within forty-eight hours of delivery) or intrapartum (at the time of cesarean section), then they are tied and cut. The failure rate for postpartum or intrapartum tubal ligation may be higher than when tubal ligation is done in the non-pregnant state.

Both sterilization methods are considered 99 percent effective. Because they can be difficult to reverse, they should be chosen by adults who are certain they do not wish to have any more biological children.

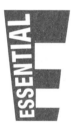

Cycle Beads are an easy way to track your fertile days when using natural family planning. A simple loop of different colored beads with a marker you move forward allows you to be aware of your most fertile times. For more information, see *www.cyclebeads.com*.

Essure is a nonsurgical sterilization method for women that involves placing small devices in each fallopian tube that cause scar tissue to grow and eventually make pregnancy impossible. It takes three months for this method to become completely effective, and another birth control method must be used in the meantime. This method is also relatively new and there will be several years of post-marketing study to evaluate effectiveness. There is also good evidence to suggest that physician experience is important in correct placement; inexperienced physicians fail to insert the fallopian devices properly in up to 14 percent of cases.

Natural Family Planning

Natural family planning, or fertility awareness, is a method of birth control that relies upon knowledge of your cycle and abstinence during fertile periods. You need to chart your basal body temperature and/or test your cervical mucous to use this accurately. This type of birth control is not as effective for women over age 35, whose cycles may be becoming irregular. Natural family planning is only 75 percent effective in preventing pregnancy.

Emergency Contraception

As of this writing, the morning-after pill, or Plan B, was set to be sold over the counter. Within three days of unprotected sex, two pills are taken twelve hours apart and prevent a fertilized egg from implanting. This is not meant to be a regular form of birth control and is 75 to 89 percent effective.

Menopause

Menopause technically occurs twelve months after a woman has her last period. This is the time in your life where your fertility ends. Menopause is not an overnight event and is something that takes months or years to complete.

These are the common symptoms of menopause:

- Change in menstrual cycle, with differing times between periods and differences in flow
- Spotting between periods
- Hot flashes
- Night sweats
- Sleeping difficulties
- Vaginal dryness and an increase in vaginal infections
- Bone density loss
- Mood shifts
- Increase in urinary incontinence
- Decrease in sexual interest

- Weight gain around the waist
- Thinning hair
- Depression
- Forgetfulness

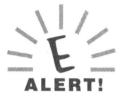

ALERT!

Autoimmune diseases—such as rheumatoid arthritis, hypothyroidism, lupus, and type 1 diabetes—in which the body attacks itself, are 2.3 times more likely to occur in women than in men. Most cases are diagnosed in women of childbearing age. Some of these diseases first appear or become worse after a pregnancy. See your health-care provider if you experience any symptoms that concern you.

Perimenopause

Perimenopause is a period of time when your body begins the transition to menopause. It can take from two to eight years, including the year after your last period. Your ovaries slowly cease functioning, and your body produces fewer amounts of certain hormones. This usually occurs between the ages of 45 and 55, but for some women it begins earlier in their thirties. Symptoms of perimenopause include the following:

- Changes in your menstrual cycle (longer or shorter, heavier or lighter, or missed periods)
- Hot flashes
- Night sweats (hot flashes while sleeping)
- Vaginal dryness
- Sleep difficulties
- Mood swings
- Increase in urinary tract infections and urinary incontinence
- Decreased sexual interest
- Increased body fat around the waist
- Memory problems

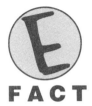

FACT

Premature menopause occurs when a woman enters menopause before age 40. Premature menopause causes the same symptoms as menopause, but they are usually stronger. Early menopause can put a woman at higher risk for bone density loss.

Birth control pills are often used to control these symptoms. It is important to note that you can still get pregnant during perimenopause, even if you're not having regular periods. Getting enough exercise, eating a healthy diet, and reducing stress can also help relieve symptoms.

Estrogen Replacement

Estrogen or hormone replacement therapy (HRT) is sometimes used to lessen the symptoms of menopause. Because your body is slowly decreasing the levels of certain hormones during menopause, replacing those hormones can offer relief of symptoms.

Women undergoing HRT are given estrogen or estrogen with progestin as supplements. HRT can reduce bone loss, vaginal dryness, night sweats, and hot flashes. The benefits of HRT must be balanced against the risks, which include blood clots, heart attacks, strokes, breast cancer, endometrial cancer, and gall bladder disease. For women who choose to use HRT upon the advice of their health-care provider, it is recommended that the smallest effective dose be used to minimize risks.

Health Risks As You Age

As women age, their risks for certain conditions and diseases increases. In general, it is best to live as healthy a life as you can, including a nutritious diet, regular exercise, and regular checkups. While the risks for the conditions described in this section do go up as you age, that does not mean you are going to experience one or any of them. Still, they are risks you should be aware of.

Breast Cancer

Breast cancer is a devastating disease that will affect 12.7 percent of women. Your risks for breast cancer increase with age. Women ages 30 to 39 have a .43 percent risk, and women ages 40 to 49 have a risk of 1.44 percent. Note that these numbers have been calculated only using white women, and each woman's risk differs based on her ethnicity, health, and family history.

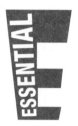

To learn your personal risk of breast cancer, use the online Breast Cancer Risk Assesssment Tool at *www.cancer.gov/bcrisktool.*

Breast cancer is often detected when a hard lump is found in the breast by the woman or her health-care provider. Mammograms are also important for breast cancer detection. Breast self-exams are no longer a recommendation because they find very few lumps and those that are found are often benign. Being familiar with your own breasts is important, though, and doing regular breast exams is not harmful or discouraged.

Other Cancers

Seventy-seven percent of all cancers are diagnosed in people over age 55, so age is a significant factor in cancer risk. Lung cancer is the leading cause of cancer death in women and becomes more likely after age 50, but the risk is highest for current or past smokers. This cancer often has no symptoms, but women should report coughing up blood to their health-care providers.

Ovarian cancer mostly occurs in women who are post-menopausal and is the fifth-highest cause of cancer death for women. Half of all ovarian cancer occurs in women who are over the age of 63. Getting a yearly pelvic exam is recommended, as is reporting bloating, pelvic pain, or abdominal changes.

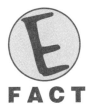

FACT

The American Cancer Society recommends that a woman should have a baseline mammogram done by age 40. Women over 40 should have a mammogram every other year and women over 50 should have one yearly. Women with a family history of breast cancer should consult their doctor about mammogram frequency and timing.

Women in their thirties and forties are at increased risk for lymphoma, which is accompanied by swollen lymph nodes, fatigue, low-grade fevers, and weight loss. Colon cancer risks increase after age 50, and all women over this age should be screened. Screening options include one of these five methods:

- Yearly fecal occult blood test or fecal immunochemical test
- Flexible sigmoidoscopy every five years
- Yearly fecal occult blood test or fecal immunochemical test and flexible sigmoidoscopy every five years
- Air contrast barium enema every five years
- Colonoscopy every ten years

Women with certain risk factors may need earlier or more frequent screening. You should consult your health-care provider to assess your risk. Report any change in bowel habits, including bleeding, to your physician.

Cervical cancer risks decrease as you become older, but those that do occur are more likely to have poor outcomes, so it is important to continue to have Pap smears. Pap smear screening should be done yearly with conventional Pap tests and every two years with liquid-based Pap tests. After age 30, women who have had three normal Pap smears in a row may have a Pap smear every two to three years, or every three years with Pap smear and human papilloma virus DNA testing.

Heart Disease

Heart disease is the leading cause of death among American women and kills 32 percent of women—almost twice as many as all cancers combined. The risk for heart disease increases with age. Cardiovascular disease, which includes heart disease as well as strokes, is responsible for 39 percent of female deaths. To reduce your risk, get your cholesterol levels checked at least once every five years and work to get them into acceptable ranges. Have your blood pressure checked regularly. Get regular exercise, and eat a healthy diet. Quit smoking and get tested for diabetes.

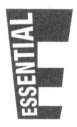

You can take an online assessment to determine your personal risk for heart disease at *http://goredforwomen.org/know_your_numbers/go_red_heart_check.html.*

Thyroiditis

Five to 7 percent of women experience postpartum hypothyroidism, or thyroiditis, in which the thyroid gland is suppressed by the autoimmune system after pregnancy. Hashimoto's thyroiditis is a similar condition, but is not linked to pregnancy. It is most common after age 40. Painless inflammation of the thyroid gland, often only detectable to an experienced physician, is often the first symptom. The disease is slow to progress and symptoms can include fatigue, constipation, hair loss, and leg cramps. A simple blood test can diagnose this, and it is easily treatable with thyroid hormone replacement. All women over age 50 should be screened for thyroid disease.

Osteoporosis

Osteoporosis is a disease involving bone loss. It is silent and painless until the point at which the disease causes a bone to break or fracture, commonly the hip or spine. Menopause results in a decrease in your body's production of estrogen, a hormone that helps control bone loss. Because of this, women going through menopause are at increased risk for osteoporosis. Women are four times more likely than men to experience osteoporosis. It is more common in Caucasian and Asian women and in women who are small boned and thin.

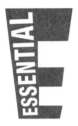

For more information about osteoporosis, contact the National Osteoporosis Foundation (online at *www.nof.org*; 202-223-2226).

Osteoporosis can be prevented. To help your bones stay healthy, get enough calcium (1000 mg per day) and vitamin D (200 IU per day), eat a healthy diet, stop smoking, and do weight-bearing exercise. Bone-density scans are recommended for all postmenopausal women between the ages of 50 and 65 who have risk factors (such as previous fractures, low body weight, smoking, or a family history). If no other risk factors are present, scans are recommended after age 65.

Type 2 Diabetes

Diabetes is a disease in which the body cannot use insulin effectively and eventually cannot make enough. The symptoms of type 2 diabetes include the following:

- Increased thirst
- Increased urination
- Increased hunger
- Fatigue
- Weight loss
- Blurred vision
- Sores that won't heal

It is important to note, however, that many individuals with type 2 diabetes may be totally asymptomatic (have no symptoms) for many years.

Screening is the only effective way to detect type 2 diabetes in its early stages before it causes additional problems.

Women over age 45 should be tested for type 2 diabetes. This should be done at least once every three years. Those who have risk factors should be tested sooner and more frequently. Risk factors include the following:

- Being overweight (body mass index over 25)
- A parent or sibling with diabetes
- Being Native American, African American, Asian American, or Hispanic
- Having had gestational diabetes or giving birth to a baby over nine pounds
- High blood pressure
- High triglycerides or low good (HDL) cholesterol
- Not exercising regularly
- Having cardiovascular disease
- Having polycystic ovarian syndrome (PCOS)

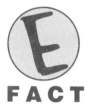

FACT

Studies show that approximately 30 to 40 percent of women who had gestational diabetes will develop type 2 diabetes within five to ten years. After ten years, the rate may be as high as 70 percent.

If you have had gestational diabetes and are contemplating future pregnancies, it is important to be screened yearly for diabetes. Screening is done with a fasting blood glucose or 75-gram glucose tolerance test. The 75-gram glucose tolerance test gives additional information and may be preferable for women contemplating pregnancy. If you screen positive for diabetes or already have type 2 diabetes, it is important that you undergo preconception diabetes care prior to becoming pregnant again. This allows screening for other complications of diabetes that may impact a future pregnancy, as well as to control blood sugars before conception to reduce the risk of birth defects. To reduce your risk of diabetes, eating a healthy diet and getting regular exercise are key. Controlling your cholesterol and blood pressure are also important.

Getting Pregnant Again

If you feel you've just begun your family and would like to have more children, you already know the ins and outs of pregnancy over 35. Doubtless you will feel more relaxed about everything should you become pregnant again.

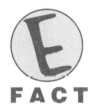

FACT

According to a 1995 report from the National Center for Health Statistics, 3.3 million women in the U.S. were at that time experiencing secondary infertility. This number is up from 2.7 million in 1988.

Before you can get pregnant again, you need to fully recover from this pregnancy. It is recommended that you space your pregnancies out with at least six months between them and an optimal spacing of twenty-four to thirty-five months. An interval shorter than six months between pregnancies is linked to having a low birth-weight baby. It is also a good idea to wait until you are done breastfeeding, since being pregnant and breastfeeding a child can be very taxing on your body.

Before getting pregnant again, take control of your weight. A recent study has shown that gaining weight between pregnancies (even as little as seven pounds, and even in women who are not overweight) can increase the risks for you and your future babies. Weight gain increases the risk for diabetes and high blood pressure as well as stillbirth, and it ups the odds of a C-section.

Secondary Infertility

Secondary infertility is the term used to describe women who have a child but experience difficulty conceiving another. If you try to conceive another child for six months with no success, it's time to see a doctor. Because fertility declines with age, the older you become, the more likely you are to experience this. Secondary infertility is just as difficult to cope with as primary infertility, but it may be more difficult to find support since women who have never had a child may have less sympathy for women experiencing secondary infertility. Secondary infertility is treated in the same way as primary infertility. Even if you've undergone fertility testing prior to your first child, you'll likely have to go through it all again because your body, and that of your partner, can change.

Appendix A

Helpful Web Sites

4Moms at Home.com
✍www.4momsathome.com
This is an excellent resource
for the stay-at-home mom.

American Baby
✍www.americanbaby.com
A site and a magazine
with great information.

American Pregnancy Association
✍www.americanpregnancy.org
This offers good cover-
age of pregnancy topics.

At Home Dad.com
✍www.athomedad.com
This is an online resource
for stay-at-home fathers.

Babycenter.com
✍www.babycenter.com
This is an excellent resource,
offering articles as well
as bulletin boards.

Babyzone.com
✍www.babyzone.com
Articles and information about
baby care and parenthood.

Baby Talk
✍www.babytalk.com
This site focuses on newborns.

Can One of You Afford to Quit?
✍www.kiplinger.com/personal
finance/tools/managing/
afford.html
Use this site's calcula-
tor to determine if you can
afford to leave your job.

Catalyst
✍www.catalystwomen.org
This site offers support and information for working women.

**Commission for the Accreditation of
Birth Centers**
✍www.birthcenters.org
This site offers information on
birth-center accreditation.

DocFinder
✍www.docboard.org
This site allows you to search
state medical board records.

Families and Work Institute
✍www.familiesandwork.org
This site offers information and
support for working parents.

Family and Home Network
✍www.familyandhome.org
This site offers information and
support for at-home parents.

**Federal and State Family
Medical Leave Laws**
✍www.dol.gov/esa/programs/
whd/state/fmla/
Use this site for important information about state and federal family leave provisions.

Fertilitext
✍www.fertilitext.org
This site offers fertility information.

Fertility Friend
✍www.fertilityfriend.com
This site offers information,
charts, and bulletin boards.

Fertility Plus
✍www.pinelandpress.com
This site is filled with helpful information, charts,
and bulletin boards.

Fit Pregnancy
✍www.fitpregnancy.com
A magazine and a Web site, this is
an excellent source of information.

International Cesarean Awareness

✍www.ican-online.org
This site offers information about birth by C-section.

Juvenile Products Manufacturers Association

✍www.jpma.org
This site offers recall and safety information about baby products.

La Leche League

✍www.lalecheleague.org
This site offers breastfeeding information and support.

Make Your Own Birth Plan

✍www.birthplan.com
Use this online tool to create a personalized birth plan.

The March of Dimes

✍www.marchofdimes.com
This site focuses on pregnancy health and the prevention of birth defects.

Maternity Center Association

✍www.maternitywise.org
This site offers information about C-sections and choosing elective C-sections.

Midlife Mommies

✍www.midlifemommies.com
This site offers information and support for older moms.

MOST

✍www.mostonline.org
This site offers support to mothers of super twins (triplets or more).

Mothers Over 40

✍www.mothersover40.com
This site offers support and information for women over 40 who are trying to become pregnant, are pregnant, or are parents.

National Association of At-Home Mothers

✍www.athomemothers.org
This site offers information and support for stay-at-home moms.

National Down Syndrome Congress

✍www.NDSCCenter.org
This site offers information about and support for Down syndrome.

National Down Syndrome Society

✍www.ndss.org
This site offers information about and support for Down syndrome.

National Organization of Mothers of Twins Club

✍www.nomotc.org
This site offers information and support for mothers of twins.

The National Women's Health Information Center

✍www.4woman.gov
This government site offers a wide range of health information meant expressly for women.

Pregnancy and Infant Loss Support

✍www.nationalshareoffice.com
This site offers information and support about miscarriage, stillbirth, and infant loss.

Resolve

✍www.resolve.org
This site offers fertility information and support.

Sidelines

✍www.sidelines.org
This site offers information and support for pregnancy bed rest.

Working Mother

✍www.workingmother.com
This is a Web site and magazine that supports working moms.

Your Plus Size Pregnancy

✍www.yourplussizepregnancy.com
This site offers support, information, and resources for plus-sized expectant moms.

Zero to Three

✍www.zerotothree.org
This site offers information about infant and toddler development.

Appendix B

Additional Resources

Organizations

American Academy of Pediatrics
141 Northwest Point Blvd.
Elk Grove Village, IL 60007
847-434-8000
✍www.aap.org

American Association of Birth Centers
3123 Gottschall Road
Perkiomenville, PA 18074
215-234-8068
✍www.birthcenters.org

American College of Nurse-Midwives
8403 Colesville Rd., Suite 1550
Silver Spring, MD 20910
✍www.acnm.org

American College of Obstetricians and Gynecologists
409 12th Street SW
P.O. Box 96920
Washington, DC 20090-6920
✍www.acog.org

The American Fertility Association
666 Fifth Avenue Suite 278
New York, NY 10103
✍www.theafa.org

Depression After Delivery
91 East Somerset Street
Raritan, NJ 08869
800-944-4773
✍www.depressionafterdelivery.com

Doulas of North America
P.O. Box 626
Jasper, IN 47547
888-788-DONA
✍www.dona.org

Family and Home Network
9493-C Silver King Court
Fairfax, VA 22031
703-352-1072
✍www.familyandhome.org

International Childbirth Educators Association
P.O. Box 20048
Minneapolis, MN 55420
952-854-8660
✍www.icea.org

International Council on Infertility Information Dissemination
P.O. Box 6836
Arlington, VA 22206
703-579-9178
✍www.inciid.org

International Lactation Consultant Association
1500 Sunday Drive, Suite 102
Raleigh, NC 27607
919-861-5577
✍www.ilca.org

Juvenile Products Manufacturers Association
17000 Commerce Parkway, Suite C
Mt. Laurel, NJ 08054
856 638-0420
✍www.jpma.org

Midwives Alliance of North America
4805 Lawrenceville Hwy
Suite 116-279
Lilburn, GA 30047
888-923-MANA (6262)
✍www.mana.org

National Association of At Home Mothers
406 E. Buchanan Ave.
Fairfield, IA 52556
✍www.athomemothers.com

National Association for Family Child Care
5202 Pinemont Drive
Salt Lake City, UT 84123
801-269-9338
www.nafcc.org

National Child Care Association
1016 Rosser Street
Conyers, GA 30012
800-543-7161
www.nccanet.org

National Down Syndrome Society
666 Broadway
New York, NY 10012
800-221-4602
www.ndss.org

National Partnership for Women & Families
1875 Connecticut Avenue, NW, Suite 710
Washington, DC 20009
202-986-2600
www.nationalpartnership.org/

National Society of Genetic Counselors
233 Canterbury Drive
Wallingford, PA 1906-6617
www.nsgc.org

The North American Registry of Midwives
5257 Rosestone Dr.
Lilburn, GA 3004
888-842-4784
www.narm.org

Parents Without Partners, Inc.
1650 South Dixie Highway, Suite 510
Boca Raton, FL 33432
561-391-8833
www.parentswithoutpartners.com

United States Breastfeeding Committee
1500 Sunday Drive, Suite 102
Raleigh, NC 27607
919-861-5589
www.usbreastfeeding.org

Waterbirth International
P.O. Box 1400
Wilsonville, OR 97070
503-673-0026
www.waterbirth.org

Women, Work!
The National Network for Women's Employment
1625 K Street NW, Suite 300
Washington, DC 20006
202-467-6346
www.womenwork.org

Books

Bouchez, Collette. *Your Perfectly Pampered Pregnancy: Beauty, Health, and Lifestyle Advice for the Modern Mother-to-Be.* (Broadway, 2004).

Brott, Armin. *The Expectant Father: Facts, Tips and Advice for Dads-to-Be.* (Abbeville Press, 2001).

Bruce, Debra Fulghum. *Making a Baby: Everything You Need to Know to Get Pregnant.*

Connolly, Maureen. *The Essential C-Section Guide: Pain Control, Healing at Home, Getting Your Body Back, and Everything Else You Need to Know About a Cesarean Birth.* (Broadway, 2004).

Douglas, Ann. *The Mother of All Pregnancy Books: The Ultimate Guide to Conception, Birth, and Everything In Between.* (John Wiley and Sons, 2002).

Goer, Henci. *The Thinking Woman's Guide to a Better Birth*. (Perigee, 1999).

Hall, Nancy. *Balancing Pregnancy and Work: How to Make the Most of the Next 9 Months on the Job*. (Rodale, 2004).

Iovine, Vicki. *The Girlfriends' Guide to Pregnancy*. (Pocket Books, 1995).

Jones, Catherine. *Eating for Pregnancy: An Essential Guide to Nutrition with Recipes for the Whole Family*. (Marlowe, 2003).

King, Michael. *Pilates for Pregnancy*. (Ulysses, 2002).

Marshall, H. *The Doula Book: How a Trained Labor Companion Can Help You Have a Shorter, Easier, and Healthier Birth*. (Perseus, 2002).

McCutcheon, Susan. *Natural Childbirth the Bradley Way*. (Plume, 1996).

Ogle, Amy. *Before Your Pregnancy: A 90-Day Guide for Couples on How to Prepare for a Healthy Conception*. (Ballantine, 2000).

Paget, Lou. *Hot Mama: The Ultimate Guide to Staying Sexy Throughout Your Pregnancy and the Months Beyond*. (Gotham Books, 2005).

Savage, Beverly. *Preparation for Birth: The Complete Guide to the Lamaze Method*. (Ballantine, 1987).

Sears, Martha. *The Pregnancy Book: Month-by-Month, Everything You Need to Know From America's Baby Experts*. (Little Brown and Company, 1997).

Sember, Brette. *Gay & Lesbian Parenting Choices: From Adopting or Using a Surrogate to Choosing the Perfect Father*. (Career Press, 2006).

Sember. Brette. *Unmarried with Children*. (Adams Media, 2007).

Sember, Brette. *Your Plus-Size Pregnancy: The Ultimate Guide for the Full-Figured Expectant Mom*. (Fort Lee, NJ: Barricade Books, 2005).

Sember, Brette. *Your Practical Pregnancy Planner: Everything You Need to Know About the Financial and Legal Aspects of Preparing for Your New Baby*. (New York, NY: McGraw-Hill, 2005).

Stone, Joanne. *The Pregnancy Bible: Your Complete Guide to Pregnancy and Early Parenthood*. (Firefly, 2003).

Weschler, Toni. *Taking Charge of Your Fertility: The Definitive Guide to Natural Birth Control, Pregnancy Achievement, and Reproductive Health*. (Quill, 2001).

Index

THE **EVERYTHING** SERIES!

BUSINESS & PERSONAL FINANCE

Everything® Accounting Book
Everything® Budgeting Book
Everything® Business Planning Book
Everything® Coaching and Mentoring Book, 2nd Ed.
Everything® Fundraising Book
Everything® Get Out of Debt Book
Everything® Grant Writing Book
Everything® Guide to Foreclosures
Everything® Guide to Personal Finance for Single Mothers
Everything® Home-Based Business Book, 2nd Ed.
Everything® Homebuying Book, 2nd Ed.
Everything® Homeselling Book, 2nd Ed.
Everything® Improve Your Credit Book
Everything® Investing Book, 2nd Ed.
Everything® Landlording Book
Everything® Leadership Book
Everything® Managing People Book, 2nd Ed.
Everything® Negotiating Book
Everything® Online Auctions Book
Everything® Online Business Book
Everything® Personal Finance Book
Everything® Personal Finance in Your 20s and 30s Book
Everything® Project Management Book
Everything® Real Estate Investing Book
Everything® Retirement Planning Book
Everything® Robert's Rules Book, $7.95
Everything® Selling Book
Everything® Start Your Own Business Book, 2nd Ed.
Everything® Wills & Estate Planning Book

COOKING

Everything® Barbecue Cookbook
Everything® Bartender's Book, 2nd Ed., $9.95
Everything® Calorie Counting Cookbook
Everything® Cheese Book
Everything® Chinese Cookbook
Everything® Classic Recipes Book
Everything® Cocktail Parties & Drinks Book
Everything® College Cookbook
Everything® Cooking for Baby and Toddler Book
Everything® Cooking for Two Cookbook
Everything® Diabetes Cookbook
Everything® Easy Gourmet Cookbook
Everything® Fondue Cookbook
Everything® Fondue Party Book
Everything® Gluten-Free Cookbook
Everything® Glycemic Index Cookbook
Everything® Grilling Cookbook
Everything® Healthy Meals in Minutes Cookbook
Everything® Holiday Cookbook

Everything® Indian Cookbook
Everything® Italian Cookbook
Everything® Low-Carb Cookbook
Everything® Low-Cholesterol Cookbook
Everything® Low-Fat High-Flavor Cookbook
Everything® Low-Salt Cookbook
Everything® Meals for a Month Cookbook
Everything® Mediterranean Cookbook
Everything® Mexican Cookbook
Everything® No Trans Fat Cookbook
Everything® One-Pot Cookbook
Everything® Pizza Cookbook
Everything® Quick and Easy 30-Minute,
        5-Ingredient Cookbook
Everything® Quick Meals Cookbook
Everything® Slow Cooker Cookbook
Everything® Slow Cooking for a Crowd Cookbook
Everything® Soup Cookbook
Everything® Stir-Fry Cookbook
Everything® Sugar-Free Cookbook
Everything® Tapas and Small Plates Cookbook
Everything® Tex-Mex Cookbook
Everything® Thai Cookbook
Everything® Vegetarian Cookbook
Everything® Wild Game Cookbook
Everything® Wine Book, 2nd Ed.

GAMES

Everything® 15-Minute Sudoku Book, $9.95
Everything® 30-Minute Sudoku Book, $9.95
Everything® Bible Crosswords Book, $9.95
Everything® Blackjack Strategy Book
Everything® Brain Strain Book, $9.95
Everything® Bridge Book
Everything® Card Games Book
Everything® Card Tricks Book, $9.95
Everything® Casino Gambling Book, 2nd Ed.
Everything® Chess Basics Book
Everything® Craps Strategy Book
Everything® Crossword and Puzzle Book
Everything® Crossword Challenge Book
Everything® Crosswords for the Beach Book, $9.95
Everything® Cryptic Crosswords Book, $9.95
Everything® Cryptograms Book, $9.95
Everything® Easy Crosswords Book
Everything® Easy Kakuro Book, $9.95
Everything® Easy Large-Print Crosswords Book
Everything® Games Book, 2nd Ed.
Everything® Giant Sudoku Book, $9.95
Everything® Kakuro Challenge Book, $9.95
Everything® Large-Print Crossword Challenge Book
Everything® Large-Print Crosswords Book
Everything® Lateral Thinking Puzzles Book, $9.95

Everything® Literary Crosswords Book, $9.95
Everything® Mazes Book
Everything® Memory Booster Puzzles Book, $9.95
Everything® Movie Crosswords Book, $9.95
Everything® Music Crosswords Book, $9.95
Everything® Online Poker Book, $12.95
Everything® Pencil Puzzles Book, $9.95
Everything® Poker Strategy Book
Everything® Pool & Billiards Book
Everything® Puzzles for Commuters Book, $9.95
Everything® Sports Crosswords Book, $9.95
Everything® Test Your IQ Book, $9.95
Everything® Texas Hold 'Em Book, $9.95
Everything® Travel Crosswords Book, $9.95
Everything® TV Crosswords Book, $9.95
Everything® Word Games Challenge Book
Everything® Word Scramble Book
Everything® Word Search Book

HEALTH

Everything® Alzheimer's Book
Everything® Diabetes Book
Everything® Health Guide to Adult Bipolar Disorder
Everything® Health Guide to Arthritis
Everything® Health Guide to Controlling Anxiety
Everything® Health Guide to Fibromyalgia
Everything® Health Guide to Menopause
Everything® Health Guide to OCD
Everything® Health Guide to PMS
Everything® Health Guide to Postpartum Care
Everything® Health Guide to Thyroid Disease
Everything® Hypnosis Book
Everything® Low Cholesterol Book
Everything® Nutrition Book
Everything® Reflexology Book
Everything® Stress Management Book

HISTORY

Everything® American Government Book
Everything® American History Book, 2nd Ed.
Everything® Civil War Book
Everything® Freemasons Book
Everything® Irish History & Heritage Book
Everything® Middle East Book
Everything® World War II Book, 2nd Ed.

HOBBIES

Everything® Candlemaking Book
Everything® Cartooning Book
Everything® Coin Collecting Book
Everything® Drawing Book

Everything® Family Tree Book, 2nd Ed.
Everything® Knitting Book
Everything® Knots Book
Everything® Photography Book
Everything® Quilting Book
Everything® Sewing Book
Everything® Soapmaking Book, 2nd Ed.
Everything® Woodworking Book

HOME IMPROVEMENT

Everything® Feng Shui Book
Everything® Feng Shui Decluttering Book, $9.95
Everything® Fix-It Book
Everything® Green Living Book
Everything® Home Decorating Book
Everything® Home Storage Solutions Book
Everything® Homebuilding Book
Everything® Organize Your Home Book, 2nd Ed.

KIDS' BOOKS

All titles are $7.95

Everything® Kids' Animal Puzzle & Activity Book
Everything® Kids' Baseball Book, 4th Ed.
Everything® Kids' Bible Trivia Book
Everything® Kids' Bugs Book
Everything® Kids' Cars and Trucks Puzzle and Activity Book
Everything® Kids' Christmas Puzzle & Activity Book
Everything® Kids' Cookbook
Everything® Kids' Crazy Puzzles Book
Everything® Kids' Dinosaurs Book
Everything® Kids' Environment Book
Everything® Kids' Fairies Puzzle and Activity Book
Everything® Kids' First Spanish Puzzle and Activity Book
Everything® Kids' Gross Cookbook
Everything® Kids' Gross Hidden Pictures Book
Everything® Kids' Gross Jokes Book
Everything® Kids' Gross Mazes Book
Everything® Kids' Gross Puzzle & Activity Book
Everything® Kids' Halloween Puzzle & Activity Book
Everything® Kids' Hidden Pictures Book
Everything® Kids' Horses Book
Everything® Kids' Joke Book
Everything® Kids' Knock Knock Book
Everything® Kids' Learning Spanish Book
Everything® Kids' Magical Science Experiments Book
Everything® Kids' Math Puzzles Book
Everything® Kids' Mazes Book
Everything® Kids' Money Book
Everything® Kids' Nature Book
Everything® Kids' Pirates Puzzle and Activity Book
Everything® Kids' Presidents Book
Everything® Kids' Princess Puzzle and Activity Book
Everything® Kids' Puzzle Book
Everything® Kids' Racecars Puzzle and Activity Book
Everything® Kids' Riddles & Brain Teasers Book
Everything® Kids' Science Experiments Book
Everything® Kids' Sharks Book

Everything® Kids' Soccer Book
Everything® Kids' Spies Puzzle and Activity Book
Everything® Kids' States Book
Everything® Kids' Travel Activity Book

KIDS' STORY BOOKS

Everything® Fairy Tales Book

LANGUAGE

Everything® Conversational Japanese Book with CD, $19.95
Everything® French Grammar Book
Everything® French Phrase Book, $9.95
Everything® French Verb Book, $9.95
Everything® German Practice Book with CD, $19.95
Everything® Inglés Book
Everything® Intermediate Spanish Book with CD, $19.95
Everything® Italian Practice Book with CD, $19.95
Everything® Learning Brazilian Portuguese Book with CD, $19.95
Everything® Learning French Book with CD, 2nd Ed., $19.95
Everything® Learning German Book
Everything® Learning Italian Book
Everything® Learning Latin Book
Everything® Learning Russian Book with CD, $19.95
Everything® Learning Spanish Book with CD, 2nd Ed., $19.95
Everything® Russian Practice Book with CD, $19.95
Everything® Sign Language Book
Everything® Spanish Grammar Book
Everything® Spanish Phrase Book, $9.95
Everything® Spanish Practice Book with CD, $19.95
Everything® Spanish Verb Book, $9.95
Everything® Speaking Mandarin Chinese Book with CD, $19.95

MUSIC

Everything® Drums Book with CD, $19.95
Everything® Guitar Book with CD, 2nd Ed., $19.95
Everything® Guitar Chords Book with CD, $19.95
Everything® Home Recording Book
Everything® Music Theory Book with CD, $19.95
Everything® Reading Music Book with CD, $19.95
Everything® Rock & Blues Guitar Book with CD, $19.95
Everything® Rock and Blues Piano Book with CD, $19.95
Everything® Songwriting Book

NEW AGE

Everything® Astrology Book, 2nd Ed.
Everything® Birthday Personology Book
Everything® Dreams Book, 2nd Ed.
Everything® Love Signs Book, $9.95
Everything® Love Spells Book, $9.95
Everything® Numerology Book
Everything® Paganism Book
Everything® Palmistry Book
Everything® Psychic Book
Everything® Reiki Book
Everything® Sex Signs Book, $9.95

Everything® Spells & Charms Book, 2nd Ed.
Everything® Tarot Book, 2nd Ed.
Everything® Toltec Wisdom Book
Everything® Wicca and Witchcraft Book

PARENTING

Everything® Baby Names Book, 2nd Ed.
Everything® Baby Shower Book, 2nd Ed.
Everything® Baby's First Year Book
Everything® Birthing Book
Everything® Breastfeeding Book
Everything® Father-to-Be Book
Everything® Father's First Year Book
Everything® Get Ready for Baby Book, 2nd Ed.
Everything® Get Your Baby to Sleep Book, $9.95
Everything® Getting Pregnant Book
Everything® Guide to Pregnancy Over 35
Everything® Guide to Raising a One-Year-Old
Everything® Guide to Raising a Two-Year-Old
Everything® Guide to Raising Adolescent Boys
Everything® Guide to Raising Adolescent Girls
Everything® Homeschooling Book
Everything® Mother's First Year Book
Everything® Parent's Guide to Childhood Illnesses
Everything® Parent's Guide to Children and Divorce
Everything® Parent's Guide to Children with ADD/ADHD
Everything® Parent's Guide to Children with Asperger's Syndrome
Everything® Parent's Guide to Children with Autism
Everything® Parent's Guide to Children with Bipolar Disorder
Everything® Parent's Guide to Children with Depression
Everything® Parent's Guide to Children with Dyslexia
Everything® Parent's Guide to Children with Juvenile Diabetes
Everything® Parent's Guide to Positive Discipline
Everything® Parent's Guide to Raising a Successful Child
Everything® Parent's Guide to Raising Boys
Everything® Parent's Guide to Raising Girls
Everything® Parent's Guide to Raising Siblings
Everything® Parent's Guide to Sensory Integration Disorder
Everything® Parent's Guide to Tantrums
Everything® Parent's Guide to the Strong-Willed Child
Everything® Parenting a Teenager Book
Everything® Potty Training Book, $9.95
Everything® Pregnancy Book, 3rd Ed.
Everything® Pregnancy Fitness Book
Everything® Pregnancy Nutrition Book
Everything® Pregnancy Organizer, 2nd Ed., $16.95
Everything® Toddler Activities Book
Everything® Toddler Book
Everything® Tween Book
Everything® Twins, Triplets, and More Book

PETS

Everything® Aquarium Book
Everything® Boxer Book
Everything® Cat Book, 2nd Ed.
Everything® Chihuahua Book

Everything® **Cooking for Dogs Book**
Everything® Dachshund Book
Everything® Dog Book
Everything® Dog Health Book
Everything® Dog Obedience Book
Everything® Dog Owner's Organizer, $16.95
Everything® Dog Training and Tricks Book
Everything® German Shepherd Book
Everything® Golden Retriever Book
Everything® Horse Book
Everything® Horse Care Book
Everything® Horseback Riding Book
Everything® Labrador Retriever Book
Everything® Poodle Book
Everything® Pug Book
Everything® Puppy Book
Everything® Rottweiler Book
Everything® Small Dogs Book
Everything® Tropical Fish Book
Everything® Yorkshire Terrier Book

REFERENCE

Everything® American Presidents Book
Everything® Blogging Book
Everything® Build Your Vocabulary Book
Everything® Car Care Book
Everything® Classical Mythology Book
Everything® Da Vinci Book
Everything® Divorce Book
Everything® Einstein Book
Everything® Enneagram Book
Everything® Etiquette Book, 2nd Ed.
Everything® **Guide to Edgar Allan Poe**
Everything® Inventions and Patents Book
Everything® Mafia Book
Everything® **Martin Luther King Jr. Book**
Everything® Philosophy Book
Everything® Pirates Book
Everything® Psychology Book

RELIGION

Everything® Angels Book
Everything® Bible Book
Everything® **Bible Study Book with CD, $19.95**
Everything® Buddhism Book
Everything® Catholicism Book
Everything® Christianity Book
Everything® Gnostic Gospels Book
Everything® History of the Bible Book
Everything® Jesus Book
Everything® Jewish History & Heritage Book
Everything® Judaism Book
Everything® Kabbalah Book
Everything® Koran Book

Everything® Mary Book
Everything® Mary Magdalene Book
Everything® Prayer Book
Everything® Saints Book, 2nd Ed.
Everything® Torah Book
Everything® Understanding Islam Book
Everything® **Women of the Bible Book**
Everything® World's Religions Book
Everything® Zen Book

SCHOOL & CAREERS

Everything® Alternative Careers Book
Everything® Career Tests Book
Everything® College Major Test Book
Everything® College Survival Book, 2nd Ed.
Everything® Cover Letter Book, 2nd Ed.
Everything® Filmmaking Book
Everything® Get-a-Job Book, 2nd Ed.
Everything® Guide to Being a Paralegal
Everything® Guide to Being a Personal Trainer
Everything® Guide to Being a Real Estate Agent
Everything® Guide to Being a Sales Rep
Everything® **Guide to Being an Event Planner**
Everything® Guide to Careers in Health Care
Everything® Guide to Careers in Law Enforcement
Everything® Guide to Government Jobs
Everything® **Guide to Starting and Running a Catering Business**
Everything® Guide to Starting and Running a Restaurant
Everything® Job Interview Book
Everything® New Nurse Book
Everything® New Teacher Book
Everything® Paying for College Book
Everything® Practice Interview Book
Everything® Resume Book, 2nd Ed.
Everything® Study Book

SELF-HELP

Everything® **Body Language Book**
Everything® Dating Book, 2nd Ed.
Everything® Great Sex Book
Everything® Self-Esteem Book
Everything® Tantric Sex Book

SPORTS & FITNESS

Everything® Easy Fitness Book
Everything® **Krav Maga for Fitness Book**
Everything® Running Book

TRAVEL

Everything® **Family Guide to Coastal Florida**
Everything® Family Guide to Cruise Vacations
Everything® Family Guide to Hawaii
Everything® Family Guide to Las Vegas, 2nd Ed.
Everything® Family Guide to Mexico
Everything® Family Guide to New York City, 2nd Ed.
Everything® Family Guide to RV Travel & Campgrounds
Everything® Family Guide to the Caribbean
Everything® **Family Guide to the Disneyland® Resort, California Adventure®, Universal Studios®, and the Anaheim Area, 2nd Ed.**
Everything® **Family Guide to the Walt Disney World Resort®, Universal Studios®, and Greater Orlando, 5th Ed.**
Everything® Family Guide to Timeshares
Everything® Family Guide to Washington D.C., 2nd Ed.

WEDDINGS

Everything® Bachelorette Party Book, $9.95
Everything® Bridesmaid Book, $9.95
Everything® Destination Wedding Book
Everything® Elopement Book, $9.95
Everything® Father of the Bride Book, $9.95
Everything® Groom Book, $9.95
Everything® Mother of the Bride Book, $9.95
Everything® Outdoor Wedding Book
Everything® Wedding Book, 3rd Ed.
Everything® Wedding Checklist, $9.95
Everything® Wedding Etiquette Book, $9.95
Everything® Wedding Organizer, 2nd Ed., $16.95
Everything® Wedding Shower Book, $9.95
Everything® Wedding Vows Book, $9.95
Everything® Wedding Workout Book
Everything® **Weddings on a Budget Book, 2nd Ed., $9.95**

WRITING

Everything® Creative Writing Book
Everything® Get Published Book, 2nd Ed.
Everything® Grammar and Style Book
Everything® Guide to Magazine Writing
Everything® Guide to Writing a Book Proposal
Everything® Guide to Writing a Novel
Everything® Guide to Writing Children's Books
Everything® Guide to Writing Copy
Everything® **Guide to Writing Graphic Novels**
Everything® Guide to Writing Research Papers
Everything® Screenwriting Book
Everything® Writing Poetry Book
Everything® Writing Well Book